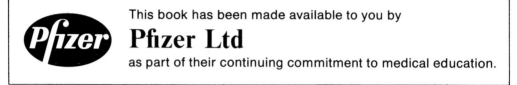

The Management of Acute Myocardial Ischaemia

Edited by

D.A. Chamberlain
Consultant Cardiologist
Royal Sussex County Hospital
Brighton, UK

D.G. Julian
Consultant Medical Director
British Heart Foundation
London, UK

and

P. Sleight
Field-Marshall Alexander
Professor of Cardiovascular Medicine
John Radcliffe Hospital
Oxford, UK

Published by Current Medical Literature Ltd, London

©1990 Current Medical Literature Ltd,
40–42 Osnaburgh Street, London NW1 3ND, UK

Printed by H Charlesworth & Co Ltd, Huddersfield, HD2 1JJ

ISBN 0 412 40150 9

List of contributors

L. Araujo
MRC Cyclotron Unit,
Hammersmith Hospital,
London, UK

M.E. Bertrand
Service de Cardiologie B et
Hemodynamique,
Hopital Cardiologique,
Lille, France

G.V.R. Born
The William Harvey Research Institute,
St Bartholomew's Hospital Medical
College,
London, UK

M.J. Buxton
Health Economics Research Group,
Brunel University,
Uxbridge, UK

R.W.F. Campbell
Department of Cardiology,
Freeman Hospital,
Newcastle upon Tyne, UK

D.A. Chamberlain
Department of Cardiology,
Royal Sussex County Hospital,
Brighton, UK

J.H. Chesebro
Mayo Clinic,
Rochester, MN, USA

S.M. Cobbe
Department of Medical Cardiology,
Royal Infirmary,
Glasgow, UK

D. Collen
Center for Thrombosis and Vascular
Research,
Katholieke Universiteit Leuven,
Leuven, Belgium

R. Collins
International Studies of Infarct
Survival,
Radcliffe Infirmary,
Oxford, UK

C. Cowan
Department of Cardiovascular Studies,
University of Leeds,
Leeds, UK

G. Davies
Cardiovascular Building,
Royal Postgraduate Medical School,
London, UK

M.J. Davies
St George's Hospital,
London, UK

D. De Bono
Department of Cardiology,
Glenfield General Hospital,
Leicester, UK

E. Falk
Institute of Forensic Medicine,
Odense University,
Odense, Denmark

J.S. Forrester
Cardiovascular Research,
Cedars-Sinai Medical Center,
Los Angeles, CA, USA

V. Fuster
Division of Cardiology,
The Mount Sinai Medical Center,
New York, NY, USA

D.J. Hearse
The Rayne Institute,
St Thomas' Hospital,
London, UK

W.S. Hillis
Department of Materia Medica,
Stobhill General Hospital,
Glasgow, UK

J. Hirsh
Department of Medicine,
McMaster University,
Hamilton, Ont, Canada

S. Holmberg
Division of Cardiology,
Sahlgrenska Hospital,
Goteborg, Sweden

J.H. Ip
Division of Cardiology,
The Mount Sinai Medical Center,
New York, NY, USA

T. Jones
Royal Postgraduate Medical School,
London, UK

D. G. Julian
British Heart Foundation,
London, UK

W. Kübler
Medizinische Universitatsklinik,
Heidelberg, West Germany

A. Leizorovicz
European Myocardial Infarction
Project,
Unite de Pharmacologie Clinique,
Hopital Neuro-Cardiologique,
Lyon, France

C. Lendon
King's College,
London, UK

A. Maseri
Cardiovascular Building,
Royal Postgraduate Medical School,
London, UK

A.L. Muir
Edinburgh Post-Graduate Board for
Medicine,
Pfizer Foundation,
Edinburgh, UK

R.M. Norris
Coronary-Care Unit,
Green Lane Hospital,
Auckland, New Zealand

M.F. Oliver
Wynn Institute for Metabolic Research,
London, UK

P.D. Richardson
Brown University,
Providence, RI, USA

A.M. Ross
Division of Cardiology,
George Washington University,
Washington, DC, USA

J.M. Rowley
King's Mill Hospital,
Mansfield, UK

R. Schröder
Universitatsklinikum Steglitz,
Freie Universitat Berlin,
Berlin, West Germany

M.L. Simoons
Thorax Centre, Erasmus University,
Rotterdam, The Netherlands

P. Sleight
Cardiac Department,
John Radcliffe Hospital,
Oxford, UK

K. Swedberg
Department of Medicine,
Gothenburg University,
Gothenburg, Sweden

G. Tognoni
Institute Mario Negri,
Milano, Italy

R. Vincent
Department of Cardiology,
Royal Sussex County Hospital,
Brighton, UK

R.G. Wilcox
University Hospital,
Queen's Medical Centre,
Nottingham, UK

Contents

3. THROMBOLYSIS

4. ADJUVANT STRATEGIES: MEDICAL INTERVENTIONS

5. ADJUVANT STRATEGIES: MECHANICAL INTERVENTIONS

6. THE FUTURE

Preface

Thrombolytic therapy has ushered in a new era in the management of myocardial infarction, but it is both the culmination of many years of research and a stimulus to fresh approaches. New applications of old approaches, such as morbid anatomy, new diagnostic techniques, such as angioscopy and PET scanning, new adjuvant therapies, and the overall strategies of management all require a critical evaluation.

The British Heart Foundation, recognizing that research in this area has reached an exciting point, organized an international conference in London in June 1989 which many of the leading workers in the field attended.

The first session dealt with the important progress in our understanding of the mechanisms involved in acute myocardial ischaemia, and the second with the newer diagnostic methods.

Although the place of thrombolysis in myocardial infarction is now assured, the conference addressed the many questions that remain to be answered. Furthermore, there is still uncertainty about the role of the various forms of adjuvant therapy — both medical and interventional — now available.

Finally, a look was taken into the future, and consideration given as to how advances in research could be translated into the most effective practice.

This volume contains the material presented at that conference and provides an overview of many of the most important topics in acute coronary disease today.

D.G. Julian
London 1990

1. THE PATHOPHYSIOLOGY OF ACUTE MYOCARDIAL ISCHAEMIA

THE PATHOLOGY OF UNSTABLE ANGINA AND MYOCARDIAL INFARCTION

E. FALK

In recent years it has become increasingly clear that thrombus formation plays a major role in acute ischaemic heart attacks [1]. A rational approach to the management of patients with acute ischaemic syndromes demands, therefore, some knowledge of the fundamental mechanisms underlying the initiation, promotion and growth of a coronary thrombus and the dynamic changes occurring during the evolution of a thrombus.

Coronary thrombosis
What happens in a coronary artery which has been diseased for years when it suddenly occludes by thrombus formation?

A postmortem coronary angiogram from a 58-year-old man who died suddenly showed a proximal intraluminal filling defect of the left anterior descending artery. Consecutive cross-sections cut at 3 mm intervals through the lesion (Fig. 1A) revealed that it was a result of acute thrombosis superimposed on a stenotic, atherosclerotic plaque. White radiographic contrast medium injected postmortem distends the vascular lumen, proximal and distal to the occlusion. In the proximal segments, the intima is thickened due to atherosclerotic changes, and a very thin cap of fibrous tissue separates the vascular lumen from the soft, fatty material in the vascular wall. At the point of occlusion, the fibrous cap has ruptured, exposing the interior of the plaque. Some plaque material is missing, probably washed away by the blood. A little further distally is one of the torn ends of the fibrous cap projecting into the lumen. The corresponding histologic section (Fig. 1B) reveals a mural thrombus at the rupture site, where thrombogenic substances in the tissue have been exposed. The thrombus at the rupture site increases to become nearly occlusive just distal to the rupture site where the stenosis is maximal. Atheromatous plaque material displaced from the interior of the plaque through the ruptured surface into the vascular lumen is found deeply embedded in the luminal thrombus (Fig. 1C). The thrombus itself consists of a granular mass of aggregating platelets, some very fine strands of fibrin, and a few erythrocytes. The main component of the thrombus is platelets.

Recapitulating, the artery suddenly thrombosed because the fibrous cap ruptured, exposing the interior of the plaque to the flowing blood. Luminal thrombus evolved at the rupture site, where thrombogenic material had been exposed, and the thrombus grew to become nearly occlusive. Atheromatous plaque material, missing from sections cut proximal to the occlusion, was found deeply embedded in the luminal thrombus, clearly indicating that plaque rupture had immediately preceded luminal thrombus formation and not *vice versa*.

Theoretically, the mechanisms underlying *fatal* and *non-fatal* thrombus formation may differ, but recent angiographic studies by Nakagawa *et al.* in Japan [2] revealed angiographic evidence of ruptured atheromatous plaque under the majority

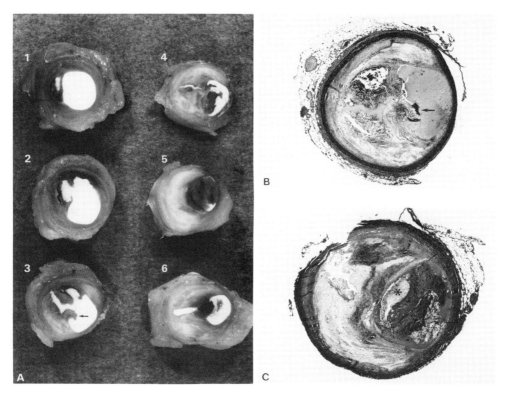

Fig. 1. Initiation of thrombosis. A. Consecutive cross sections cut at 2 mm intervals through a thrombosed coronary artery (white radiographic contrast medium is seen in the non-thrombosed vascular lumen). The thin fibrous cap separating the fatty 'gruel' from the lumen has ruptured (sections nos. 2, 3 and 4), exposing subendothelial tissue. B. Microscopic examination of section no. 3 revealing mural thrombosis at one of the free ends of the ruptured cap which projects into the lumen (arrow). C. Just distal to the rupture (section no. 5) the lumen is nearly totally occluded by aggregating platelets, and a big fragment of the ruptured fibrous cap (big asterisk) and extruded plaque material with cholesterol crystals (small asterisk) are seen within the luminal thrombosis, clearly indicating that plaque rupture has preceded luminal thrombus formation.

of coronary thrombi. So, plaque rupture seems to play a major role in both fatal and non-fatal coronary thromboses. However, rupture of the plaque surface does not always cause luminal thrombosis: rupture may result in haemorrhage from the lumen into the plaque without gross evidence of thrombosis at the rupture site; alternatively, in addition to haemorrhage into the soft lipid material a non-occlusive luminal thrombosis may evolve with consequent rapid progression of the stenosis. Davies *et al.* [3] describe such a haemorrhage superficially located into the plaque as an 'intra-intimal thrombus', because it is often in continuity with an intraluminal thrombus and, like an intraluminal thrombus, it consists of many aggregating platelets.

Microscopic examination of coronary thrombi and ruptured plaques reveals that the degree of pre-existing stenosis at the rupture site is one of the main determinants of outcome [4]. The greater the pre-existing stenosis at the rupture site, the greater the risk of thrombus formation when plaque rupture occurs. It seems reasonable to conclude that a stenosis causing rapid flow promotes arterial thrombus formation. This is in agreement with experimental studies showing that rapid flow and high shear forces activate platelets and stimulate platelet aggregation [5]. It also fits the clinical situation, where a severe stenosis often remains after otherwise successful thrombolysis. Rethrombosis following thrombolysis appears to be related to residual stenosis — the more severe the residual stenosis, the higher the risk of rethrombosis [6]. Recent clinical trials suggest that this association may, however, be eliminated by aspirin and/or heparin treatment [7].

Severe pre-existing stenosis is not always apparent angiographically following thrombolysis [8], however, and a severe stenosis or a ruptured plaque surface is not always found at postmortem examination, so other factors may also be important. In addition to the *severity of stenosis* and the *nature and extent of exposed thrombogenic material*, the actual *thrombotic/thrombolytic equilibrium* seems to be a major determinant of coronary thrombosis. It is possible to modify this equilibrium with aspirin, heparin and plasminogen activators, with beneficial effects on prognosis [9,10]. Coronary spasm may contribute to the dynamic occlusion before, during and after infarction [11], but the significance of spasm in the pathogenesis of a coronary thrombus remains speculative. Coronary spasm has usually been held responsible for what has been called 'infarction with normal coronary arteries', but a recent study suggests that thrombus formation also plays a role in these cases [12].

If plaque rupture leads to luminal thrombosis, it seldom does so abruptly in a single event. Usually a coronary thrombus is layered, indicating an episodic growth [13]. Fig. 2 shows a cross-section through an occluded coronary artery, obtained postmortem. The thrombus is layered, indicating episodic growth over an extended period of time. The most recent portion, located centrally, consists predominantly of aggregated platelets, while the older part of the thrombus, near, and partly incor-

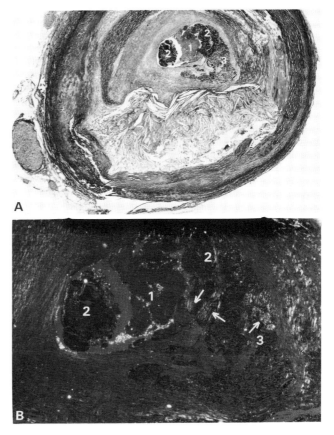

Fig. 2. Episodic thrombus formation. Most coronary thrombi have a layered structure indicating episodic growth by repeated mural deposits. In this case three layers (1-3) are clearly identified. The most recent part located centrally (1) consists predominantly of aggregated platelets, while the older parts nearer the vessel wall are homogenous (2 and 3), and partly birefringent (arrows in B, polarization microscopy), due to the presence of polymerized fibrin. Fibrin probably stabilizes the primary platelet thrombosis.

porated into the vessel wall, is homogeneous without structure. Polarization microscopy of the histologic section reveals birefringency of the older, homogeneous part of the thrombus, indicating the presence of polymerized fibrin. The most recent part of the thrombus is almost totally devoid of fibrin at the light microscopic level, consisting of aggregated platelets. This is in agreement with experimental studies on arterial thrombosis which show that the primary flow obstruction is due to platelet aggregation. This platelet thrombus, however, seems to be very fragile and unstable, and it may easily be washed away unless secondarily it is infiltrated and stabilized by fibrin [14]. Consequently, the younger the thrombus the easier it lyses [15]. The involvement of both platelets and fibrin in coronary thrombus formation implies potential benefits from the use of both antiplatelet agents and anticoagulants.

During the evolution of a coronary thrombus, episodic growth seems to alternate with thrombus fragmentation, disintegration and peripheral embolization, as indicated by the frequent finding of thromboemboli in the myocardium downstream from evolving coronary thrombi [13,16]. Such microemboli may be associated with micro-infarcts.

Unstable angina and acute myocardial infarction
Haemodynamic monitoring of patients with unstable angina has shown that transient reduction in coronary blood flow, rather than increase in myocardial oxygen demand, is usually the principal underlying mechanism in rest angina, and the concept of dynamic (as opposed to fixed) coronary stenosis has been introduced. A dynamic thrombotic process could underlie the dynamic flow obstruction of unstable angina and, indeed, seems to do so, at least in the great majority of cases with the worst prognosis — the cases culminating in infarction or sudden death [13,17].

The number and degree of stenoses have been reported to be similar in stable and unstable angina, despite the poorer prognosis of the latter. Hence, the difference between stable and unstable angina could be *qualitative* — an intact versus a disrupted plaque surface — rather than *quantitative* — the number and degree of stenoses. Accordingly, unstable angina seems to be associated with irregular stenoses which progress rapidly, often accompanied by luminal thrombosis and enhanced vasoreactivity which may cause spasm [1]. These phenomena may be accounted for by a ruptured plaque surface with variable degree of haemorrhage into the plaque and luminal thrombosis: rapid progression of the stenosis ensues, with a risk of progression to total vascular occlusion and, ultimately, infarction or sudden death. A concomitant vasospastic phenomenon could be initiated by vasoactive substances liberated from platelets at the rupture site, or could be due to the disruptive intimal haemorrhage which may reach the base of the plaque and come into close contact with smooth muscle cells in the media. It seems clear that such a mechanism — a ruptured plaque surface with a superimposed dynamic thrombosis with or without concomitant vasospasm — underlies the great majority of acute ischaemic syndromes, including unstable angina, non-Q-wave infarction (formerly called subendocardial infarction) and Q-wave infarction (formerly called transmural infarction) [18]. The clinical syndrome observed, and its outcome, depends on the duration and severity of ischaemia: whether the flow obstruction is sub-total or total, transient or persistent — or modified by collateral flow.

Infarct size
The three main determinants of infarct size are: 1) the size of the area at risk; 2) the severity and duration of ischaemia; and 3) the vulnerability of the myocardium [19].

4

The first two factors are the most important. Lee and co-workers showed that infarct size is linearly related to the size of the vascular bed at risk [20]. The extent of the at-risk vascular bed in turn depends entirely on the coronary anatomy and the site of the coronary occlusion. Fig. 3 shows the 'risk area' associated with an occlusion proximal in the left anterior descending artery and for comparison the area at risk associated with an occlusion distal in the same vessel. In the first case, occlusion may give rise to extensive infarction involving most of the septum and the antero-lateral wall of the left ventricle; this may not occur if the occlusion is located distally. 'Risk areas' associated with occlusion in the left anterior descending artery are usually greater than 'risk areas' associated with occlusion in the circumflex artery or the right coronary artery. Consequently, the treatment gain may be much greater, and more easily obtained, in anterior infarction than in posterior or inferior infarction, because much more myocardium is at risk.

Following permanent coronary occlusion in dogs, irreversible ischaemic damage occurs first in the subendocardial myocardium and then extends through the myocardium to become nearly transmural in the course of three to six hours [21]. The rate of progression depends on the severity of ischaemia. Good collateral function and timely reperfusion may save myocardium at risk. Progression probably follows a similar course in humans but the timespan may be much longer, depending on the dynamic nature of the coronary occlusion and collaterals [22]. In dogs occlusion is permanent, but in humans coronary thrombus formation is dynamic and may be accompanied by vasospasm. In addition, there is probably better collateral flow in most human subjects. Human collaterals are located epicardially, on the surface of

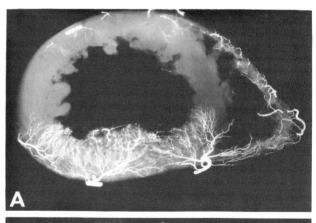

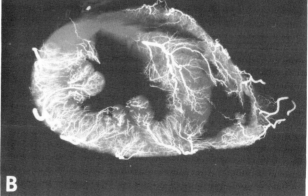

Fig. 3. Area at risk of infarction. The size of the 'risk area' depends on the coronary anatomy (given by nature) and the site of the coronary occlusion. An occlusion proximal in the left anterior descending coronary artery is associated with a much greater 'risk area' (A) than an occlusion distal in the same vessel after the takeoff of diagonal and septal branches (B) — and, consequently, may give rise to more extensive infarction.

the heart and, unlike in the dog, human collaterals are also situated intramurally and subendocardially, forming a subendocardial plexus [23].

The main determinant of available collateral flow in cases of sudden coronary occlusion seems to be the degree of the pre-existing atherosclerotic stenosis [24]. The greater this is, the greater the extent of collateral flow. The significance of this collateral flow is evident: 10% of patients with rest angina have a totally occluded coronary artery but no definite infarction because of well developed collateral circulation [25]; 25% of patients with non-Q-wave infarction have a totally occluded artery at the time of acute angiography, increasing to 40% of patients in the course of a few days [26], but due to parallel increases in collateral flow a considerable amount of myocardium is salvaged; in Q-wave infarction, 90% of patients initially have a totally occluded coronary artery and many experience a relatively extensive infarction due to poor collateral circulation [27]. Thus, collateral supply may preserve myocardium at risk.

Thrombus propagation

If the primary platelet thrombus at the rupture site occludes the lumen totally, blood proximal and distal to the occlusion may stagnate and coagulate, resulting in secondary stagnation thrombosis. Proximal propagation of the secondary stagnation thrombus may pass major side-branches without causing occlusion (Fig. 4), so proximal thrombus propagation cannot explain the phenomenon of infarct extension or

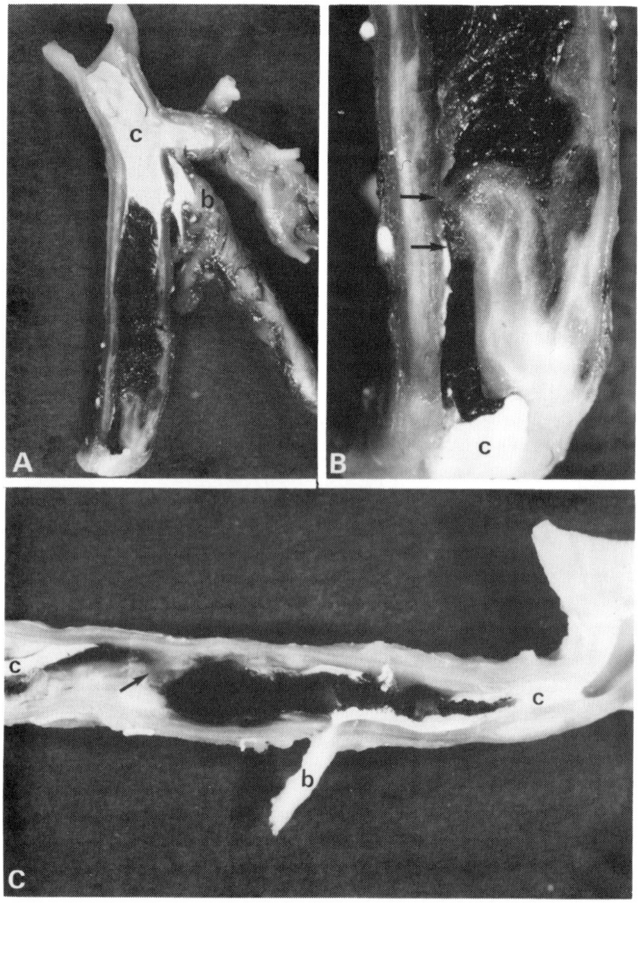

Fig. 4. Upstream thrombus propagation. A red stagnation thrombosis may form secondarily to the reduced flow caused by the primary 'white' platelet thrombosis (arrows). A,B. The red stagnation thrombosis is often impressive while the primary white thrombosis may be hard to find. C. Upstream thrombus propagation may extend beyond side-branches as a non-occlusive thrombosis, but major side-branches are not occluded by up-stream thrombus propagation.
b = side-branches;
c = contrast medium.

re-infarction. Conversely, downstream thrombus propagation may occlude side-branches (Fig. 5). The significance of this phenomenon is uncertain. Theoretically it may impede collateral flow, but probably downstream thrombus propagation only occurs if there is no significant collateral flow. Extensive downstream thrombus formation due to stagnation may, however, explain why it is not possible to re-open all occluded coronary arteries during evolving myocardial infarction. Extensive stagnation thrombosis may be very hard to lyse.

Conclusion

1) Most coronary thrombi are *initiated by rupture* of the plaque surface causing platelet aggregation where thrombogenic subendothelial tissue has been exposed. About half of all coronary thrombi contain atheromatous material displaced from the interior of the plaque into the lumen, where it is found often deeply buried in the luminal thrombus, clearly indicating that plaque rupture has preceded luminal thrombus formation and not *vice versa*.

2) *Stenoses* causing rapid flow rather than stasis seem to *promote* platelet aggregation and arterial thrombus formation. The severity of the pre-existing stenosis at the rupture site seems to be one of the main determinants of whether plaque rupture causes a small, non-occlusive thrombus or an occlusive thrombus.

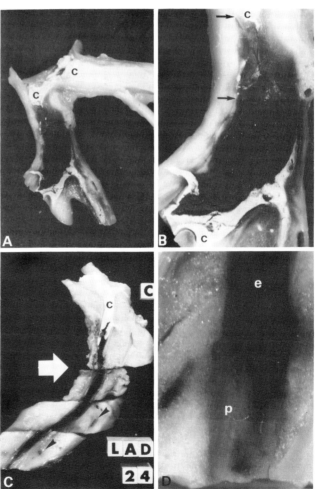

Fig. 5. Downstream thrombus propagation. A,B. The primary (white) thrombosis is just perceptible within and distal to the stenosis (between the arrows) causing flow cessation with a secondarily formed red stagnation thrombosis propagating downstream without side-branch occlusion. **C.** A primary (white) thrombosis at a severe stenosis (arrow) with extensive thrombus propagation. Major side-branches are occluded downstream (arrow heads), but the significance of this is uncertain. **D.** Occlusion at arrow in C at higher magnification showing the primary white thrombosis (p = platelets) with adjacent red stagnation thrombosis (e = erythrocytes). c = contrast medium.

7

3)   Coronary thrombus formation seems to be a *dynamic process* whereby recurrent thrombus formation alternates with fragmentation and peripheral embolization.

4)   Platelets seem to be responsible for the primary flow obstruction, but such platelet thrombi are probably very fragile and unstable and may easily be washed away unless secondarily infiltrated and stabilized by fibrin. Hence, both *platelets and fibrin* seem to play a role in coronary thrombus formation.

References

[1]   Falk E.
      Morphologic features of unstable athero-thrombotic plaques underlying acute coronary syndromes.
      Am J Cardiol 1989; **63**: 114E–120E.
[2]   Nakagawa S, Hanada Y, Koiwaya Y, Tanaka K.
      Angiographic features in the infarct-related artery after intracoronary urokinase followed by prolonged anticoagulation. Role of ruptured atheromatous plaque and adherent thrombus in acute myocardial infarction *in vivo*.
      Circulation 1988; **78**: 1335–44.
[3]   Davies MJ, Thomas AC.
      Plaque fissuring — the cause of acute myocardial infarction, sudden ischaemic death, and crescendo angina.
      Br Heart J 1985; **53**: 363–73.
[4]   Falk E.
      Plaque rupture with severe pre-existing stenosis precipitating coronary thrombosis. Characteristics of coronary atherosclerotic plaques underlying fatal occlusive thrombi.
      Br Heart J 1983; **50**: 127–34.
[5]   Badimon L, Badimon J-J, Galvez A, Chesebro JH, Fuster V.
      Influence of arterial damage and wall shear rate on platelet deposition. *Ex vivo* study in a swine model.
      Arteriosclerosis 1986; **6**: 312–20.
[6]   Harrison DG, Ferguson DW, Collins SM, et al.
      Rethrombosis after reperfusion with streptokinase: importance of geometry of residual lesions.
      Circulation 1984; **69**: 991–9.
[7]   Wall TC, Mark DB, Califf RM, et al.
      Prediction of early recurrent myocardial ischemia and coronary reocclusion after successful thrombolysis: a qualitative and quantitative angiographic study.
      Am J Cardiol 1989; **63**: 423–8.
[8]   Hackett D, Davies G, Maseri A.
      Pre-existing coronary stenoses in patients with first myocardial infarction are not necessarily severe.
      Eur Heart J 1988; **9**: 1317–23.

[9]   Théroux P, Ouimet H, McCans J, et al.
      Aspirin, heparin, or both to treat acute unstable angina.
      N Engl J Med 1988; **319**: 1105–11.
[10] ISIS-2.
      Randomised trial of intravenous streptokinase, oral aspirin, both, or neither among 17 187 cases of suspected acute myocardial infarction.
      Lancet 1988; **ii**: 349–60.
[11] Hackett D, Davies G, Chierchia S, Maseri A.
      Intermittent coronary occlusion in acute myocardial infarction. Value of combined thrombolytic and vasodilator therapy.
      N Engl J Med 1987; **317**: 1055–9.
[12] Rapold HJ, Haeberli A, Kuemmerli H, Weiss M, Baur HR, Straub WP.
      Fibrin formation and platelet activation in patients with myocardial infarction and normal coronary arteries.
      Eur Heart J 1989; **10**: 323–33.
[13] Falk E.
      Unstable angina with fatal outcome: dynamic coronary thrombosis leading to infarction and/or sudden death. Autopsy evidence of recurrent mural thrombosis with peripheral embolization culminating in total vascular occlusion.
      Circulation 1985; **71**: 699–708.
[14] Mustard JF, Packham MA, Kinlough-Rathbone RL.
      Mechanisms in thrombosis. In: Bloom AL, Thomas DP, eds. *Haemostasis and thrombosis.* Edinburgh, London, Melbourne, New York: Churchill Livingstone 1987; chapter 37.
[15] Topol EJ, Bates ER, Walton JA, et al.
      Community hospital administration of intravenous tissue plasminogen activator in acute myocardial infarction: improved timing, thrombolytic efficacy and ventricular function.
      J Am Coll Cardiol 1987; **10**: 1173–7.
[16] Davies MJ, Thomas AC, Knapman PA, Hangartner JR.
      Intramyocardial platelet aggregation in patients with unstable angina suffering sudden ischemic cardiac death.
      Circulation 1986; **73**: 418–27.

[17] Freeman MR, Williams AE, Chisholm RJ, Armstrong PW.
Intracoronary thrombus and complex morphology in unstable angina. Relation to timing of angiography and in-hospital cardiac events.
Circulation 1989; **80:** 17-23.

[18] Fuster V, Badimon L, Cohen M, Ambrose JA, Badimon JJ, Chesebro J.
Insights into the pathogenesis of acute ischemic syndromes.
Circulation 1988; **77:** 1213-20.

[19] Reimer KA, Jennings RB, Cobb FR, *et al.*
Animal models for protecting ischemic myocardium: results of the NHLBI Cooperative Study. Comparison of unconscious and conscious dog models.
Circ Res 1985; **56:** 651-65.

[20] Lee JT, Ideker RE, Reimer KA.
Myocardial infarct size and location in relation to the coronary vascular bed at risk in man.
Circulation 1981; **64:** 526-34.

[21] Reimer KA, Jennings RB.
The "wavefront phenomenon" of myocardial ischemic cell death. II. Transmural progression of necrosis within the framework of ischemic bed size (myocardium at risk) and collateral flow.
Lab Invest 1979; **40:** 633-44.

[22] Rentrop KP, Feit F, Sherman W, *et al.*
Late thrombolytic therapy preserves left ventricular function in patients with collateralized total coronary occlusion: primary end point findings of the second Mount Sinai-New York University Reperfusion Trial.
J Am Coll Cardiol 1989; **14:** 58-64.

[23] Fulton WFM.
The dynamic factor in enlargement of coronary arterial anastomoses, and paradoxical changes in the subendocardial plexus.
Br Heart J 1964; **26:** 39-50.

[24] Cohen M, Sherman W, Rentrop KP, Gorlin R.
Determinants of collateral filling observed during sudden controlled coronary artery occlusion in human subjects.
J Am Coll Cardiol 1989; **13:** 297-303.

[25] de Zwaan C, Bär FW, Janssen JHA, *et al.*
Angiographic and clinical characteristics of patients with unstable angina showing an ECG pattern indicating clinical narrowing of the proximal LAD coronary artery.
Am Heart J 1989; **117:** 657-65.

[26] DeWood MA, Stifter WF, Simpson CS, *et al.*
Coronary arteriographic findings soon after non-Q-wave myocardial infarction.
N Engl J Med 1986; **315:** 417-23.

[27] DeWood MA, Spores J, Notske R, *et al.*
Prevalence of total coronary occlusion during the early hours of transmural myocardial infarction.
N Engl J Med 1980; **303:** 897-902.

PATHOGENESIS OF FISSURING IN HUMAN ATHEROSCLEROTIC PLAQUES

C. LENDON, M.J. DAVIES, P.D. RICHARDSON, G.V.R. BORN

The following report results from a continuing collaboration between Professor Michael Davies of St George's Hospital, London; Professor Peter Richardson, Brown University, Providence, Rhode Island; and myself at the William Harvey Research Institute, St Bartholomew's Hospital Medical College, London, together with Corinne Lendon, a graduate student of King's College, London.

Plaque fissuring

Given that the primary event in most cases of coronary thrombosis is the development of cracks or fissures in atheromatous plaques, it is clearly important to establish what causes such fissuring. This is obviously a complex problem but, as a starting point, an analogy was suggested [1] between what happens in a fissuring plaque and what happens in the process known as fatigue failure. Fatigue failure is a sudden structural change affecting metallic or plastic materials which are subjected to continuously variable forces over long periods of time. The structural change may be disastrous, such as fissuring of a bridge support [1]. The situation in a coronary artery is, of course, much more complex, but similarities do exist. The heart keeps pumping blood through the coronaries, thereby generating continuously variable stresses in the vessel walls; in these circumstances, it is conceivable that a minute weak point in a hardened plaque might develop into a fissure, exactly as in fatigue failure. This is necessarily a much over-simplified picture, but it does provide a starting point for appropriately sophisticated investigations of how the mechanical properties of human postmortem plaques might be determined by their cellular and biochemical make-up and of how particular kinds of plaque structure might account for their rupture.

Computer model of stress distribution
Over the past two years Peter Richardson has developed an elegant computer model which can be programmed to imitate, on the basis of reasonable assumptions, the situation in an artery wall; for example, entries can be made for vessel stiffnesses, the forces that act on the vessel, weak or potentially weak areas such as lipid plaques, and so on. When the program is adapted to introduce a small irregularity, akin to an intimal fissure, into the model of the vessel wall, stress in the wall is greatly increased at and around that fissure [2]. This particular result is certainly compatible with the fatigue-failure analogy; nevertheless, that might be too primitive a picture of what is certainly a very complicated pathological process.

Perhaps more important is that the computer model has shown the stress distribution in and around plaque caps in situations akin to real life, in which there is a lipid pool covered by a plaque cap [2]. There is very great concentration of circumferential stress just at the edge of the lipid pool, falling away a little into the cap. This suggests that, other things being equal, the primary force-determining feature is a concentration of stress at the edges of a plaque cap. The question that immediately arises is whether this corresponds to the distribution of fissures or ruptures demonstrable in coronary arteries postmortem. Professor Davies' results do indeed show that about 50% of fissures occur at or near the point where the plaque cap joins the apparently normal wall, in reasonable agreement with the computer model. A further 30% of fissures are distributed along the rest of the plaque cap. This analysis, which is progressing, considers only force distribution, which is undoubtedly just one of several factors that determine fissuring of plaques.

Mechanical properties of plaques
In a related investigation we have been sampling plaques obtained postmortem from human aortae within the first few hours after death to determine mechanical and biochemical properties of plaques relevant to fissuring. Aortae rather than coronary arteries are used because of the amount of material required. Samples about 4 mm x 1-2 mm in size taken from the centre of a plaque cap are compared with those from the periphery of the cap and with nearby, apparently normal intima. The samples are inserted into a device, first devised by Peter Richardson and then modified by us, in which slow and continuous stretch is applied to the ends of the pieces until they break, providing a crude indication of mechanical properties. Interestingly, Corinne Lendon has noted that the base of the fibrous cap quite often has some tough cholesterol-rich material attached to it which is quite hard to dissect away. The mechanical

properties of plaques which fissured pathologically during life are compared with closely similar non-fissured plaques. The results show that, compared to samples from peripheral areas of the plaques and normal intima, stress at the point of fracture is significantly lower in samples taken from the central portions of plaques which fissured antemortem. Stress at the point of fracture in these samples is also significantly lower than in corresponding material from unfissured plaques. These results suggest that plaques that rupture pathologically have different mechanical properties which cause them to break at lower levels of stress.

Biochemical properties of plaques

Having demonstrated that fissured plaque caps actually do break more easily, how does this relate to their biochemical properties? Determinations of hydroxyproline indicate that, on a dry weight basis, samples taken from the centre of fissured plaques contain less collagen than samples from the periphery of such plaques, from adjacent normal intima, or from non-fissured plaques. Similar findings were made for total sulphated glycosaminoglycans.

We conclude that particular plaque configurations concentrate stress on the caps, mostly at their junctions with the normal vessel wall. Moreover, the fracture stress of the centre of a fissured plaque is lower than that of the plaque periphery and neighbouring normal intima, and this is associated with lower concentrations of collagen and sulphated glycosaminoglycans in the central areas. It seems, therefore, that deficiency or degradation of connective tissue matrix predispose plaques with vulnerable configurations to fissure.

What might be the cause of such degradation or deficiency of connective tissue? It has been suggested that macrophages may be involved in some way, and Michael Davies has produced evidence to support this belief. Highly specific antibody staining has been used to count macrophages in areas close to the fissures in fissured plaques, in areas of these plaques distant from sites of fissuring, and in unfissured plaques. The results of these comparisons show that plaques which have ulcerated or fissured have significantly more macrophages in their caps than are present in the caps of non-ulcerated plaques; and that neighbouring intima contains very few macrophages. These results are consistent with the diminished stress at fracture. One obvious line of thought that follows from our observations is that the macrophages become foam cells which degenerate. The necrotic cells release proteolytic enzymes which break down the connective tissues, thereby weakening the plaques and predisposing them to fissuring.

A final comment on the possible role of calcium. We know, particularly from the work of A Fleckenstein and G Fleckenstein-Grün, that the calcium content of artery walls increases with age and is also increased in hypertensives, in diabetics and apparently also in people who smoke. We have not yet analysed our plaque samples for calcium, but intuitively one would expect plaques with more calcium to be harder and more prone to the development of minor faults which may progress to fissure. These possibilities remain to be systematically investigated.

References

[1] Born GVR.
Arterial thrombosis and its prevention. In: Haydase S, Murao S, eds. *Proc. VIII World Congress of Cardiology, Tokyo.* Amsterdam: Excerpta Medica, 1979.

[2] Richardson PD, Davies MJ, Born GVR.
Influence of plaque configuration and stress distribution on fissuring of coronary atherosclerotic plaques.
Lancet 1989; **ii**: 941–4.

PLAQUE DISRUPTION AND THROMBOSIS IN ACUTE ISCHAEMIC SYNDROMES

V. FUSTER, J.H. IP, J.H. CHESEBRO

Pathological studies [1,2] of patients who died suddenly, or shortly after an episode of unstable angina or myocardial infarction, have clearly shown that fissuring or rupture of an atherosclerotic plaque in the coronary arteries plays a fundamental role in the pathogenesis of the acute ischaemic syndromes. Disrupted atherosclerotic plaques are commonly associated with formation of mural or occlusive thrombi, usually anchored to fissures in the ruptured or ulcerated plaques. In addition, emerging evidence suggests that plaque rupture, thrombosis and fibrous organization are also important in the progression of atherosclerosis in asymptomatic patients and those with stable angina. This review will discuss the emerging concepts related to: (1) the pathogenesis of atherosclerotic plaque rupture; (2) development of coronary thrombosis; (3) the pathophysiology of the acute ischaemic syndromes based on the above concepts, and (4) avenues for future therapeutic intervention and research. It should be emphasized that our understanding of this area of cardiology is rapidly evolving and, therefore, the following ideas should be considered only as proposals subject to continuous revision and change.

Atherosclerotic plaque rupture

The process of atherosclerotic plaque rupture has been known for many years [3-6]. More recent angiographic, angioscopic and pathologic studies [1,2,7-11] have clearly established an association between plaque fissuring or ulceration and the development of unstable angina, acute myocardial infarction and sudden ischaemic death. The anatomic and physiologic characteristics of ruptured plaques, the ability to identify and predict which lesions are prone to rupture, and measures aimed at reversal of this pathologic process are areas currently being explored by many investigators around the world. In this section, four concepts will be analysed: (a) rupture of small atherosclerotic plaques; (b) lipid rich plaques; (c) the roles of macrophages, and (d) effects of stress on plaque rupture.

a) Rupture of small plaques

The severity of coronary artery stenosis and the number of diseased vessels has to be known to assess future cardiac mortality and morbidity. Only over the last few years, has it become apparent that coronary lesions with less severe angiographic disease are associated with significant progression to severe stenosis or total occlusion, and that they may account for up to two-thirds of patients who develop unstable angina or acute myocardial infarction (Table 1) [12-15]. A study [13] from our laboratory in patients with unstable angina who underwent two sequential angiograms revealed that 72% of the lesions that showed progression had <50% stenosis on the first angiogram. Analysis of the morphology of coronary lesions that progressed to less than occlusion, revealed the presence of eccentric lesions with a narrowed neck and overhanging edges or scalloped border in 71% of cases. Lesions with this particular morphology are thought to represent plaque disruption with or without a partially occlusive thrombus [12]. Indeed, post-mortem angiographic studies [10] have shown that eccentric lesions with irregular borders commonly represent plaque rupture or

Table 1. Severity of coronary disease on initial angiogram in patients with subsequent ischaemic coronary events.

Disease [ref]	No. of patients	Initial stenosis (%)		
		<50	50-70	>70
Unstable angina [13]	25	72	16	12
Myocardial infarction [14]	23	48	30	22
Myocardial infarction [15]	29	66	31	3
Myocardial infarction [16]	32	32	53	15

haemorrhage, or superimposed partially occluding or recanalized thrombus.

Over the last two years, two studies addressing the issue of angiographic progression of coronary disease in patients with myocardial infarction have been published [14,15]. Ambrose *et al.* [14] found that, on the initial angiogram, the lesion responsible for the infarction had <50% stenosis in one-half of cases and <70% stenosis in over two-thirds. Similarly, Little and co-workers [15] reported that the artery that subsequently occluded had only mild stenosis (<50%) on the first angiogram in two-thirds of patients, and <70% stenosis in the vast majority of cases. Moreover, in only one-third of patients was the infarction that occurred due to occlusion of the artery with the most severe stenosis. When these studies are analysed together, it is apparent that lesions presumably responsible for the acute ischaemic events (unstable angina or myocardial infarction) are associated with only mild to moderate stenosis in a substantial number of patients at the time of first evaluation. Accordingly, Brown et al. [16] using highly magnified angiographic images of coronary arteries during streptokinase infusion for acute myocardial infarction, found that the original lesion responsible for the infarction had <60% stenosis in two-thirds of patients (Table 1).

It should be emphasized that, even though angiography is considered as the 'gold-standard' in the evaluation of coronary anatomy, several studies have concluded that this method may underestimate the severity of coronary atherosclerosis [17,18]. At post-mortem evaluation, Glagov *et al.* [18] found that coronary arteries enlarged in relation to the presence of atherosclerosis; consequently, the luminal area, as seen angiographically, may be preserved despite extensive disease of the vessel.

Therefore, two important issues need to be considered in the evaluation of patients with coronary disease. First, angiography is helpful as a marker of the severity of coronary disease but cannot accurately predict the site of future coronary occlusion since acute ischaemic events result from disruption of only mild to moderate stenotic lesions in a substantial proportion of patients. Second, angiography may underestimate the extent and severity of atherosclerotic involvement of coronary arteries.

b) Lipid rich plaques
Pathologic studies by Davies and Thomas [1] have revealed that atherosclerotic plaques are commonly composed of a crescentic mass of lipids, separated from the vessel lumen by a fibrous cap. Plaques that undergo disruption tend to be soft, with a high concentration of cholesterol and its esters. Thinning of the fibrous cap overlying the lipid core probably precedes its rupture [1]. Recent findings from the same laboratory [19] revealed that a pool of extracellular lipid within the intima, into which the fissure extended, was present in the majority of cases, and tears commonly developed at the junction of the cap with the normal vessel. In addition, a particular configuration of

the plaque, in which the lipid pool was situated eccentrically, was most commonly associated with fissuring [19,20].

Increased shear rate in the area of stenosis (as will be discussed later), acute changes in coronary pressure and tone, and bending and twisting of an artery during each heart contraction, perhaps contribute to plaque rupture, particularly when the plaques are soft and fatty [21]. In this context, when aortas of pigs with spontaneous or diet-induced atherosclerosis were analysed [22,23], we observed extensive plaque formation and ulceration in areas of lipid accumulation, as assessed by Evans blue dye staining (unpublished report).

c) Role of macrophages
The role of macrophages in atherogenesis has been recently reviewed [24,25]. In summary, macrophages participate in the uptake and metabolism of lipids, which appear to be crucial to the development of fatty streaks and advanced atherosclerotic plaques. In addition, macrophages may contribute to atherogenesis by other mechanisms including: enhancement of transport and oxidation of low-density lipoprotein (LDL), secretion of mitogen(s) which lead to proliferation of smooth muscle cell, and stimulation of plaque neo-vascularization. Most importantly, macrophages can release proteases (elastase and collagenase) which, together with the generation of toxic products (free radicals, products of lipid oxidation), may facilitate plaque rupture or vessel wall damage [25]. Indeed, histologic specimens of atherosclerotic plaques leading to thrombosis have disclosed the presence of macrophages infiltrating the cap of atherosclerotic plaques [19].

d) Effects of stress on plaque rupture
Alterations in stress within the plaque or in the circulatory system may be important in the development of atherosclerotic plaque rupture. Davies and co-workers [19,20] analysed atherosclerotic coronary plaques of patients who died of ischaemic heart disease. They found that a segmental lipid pool within the intima was commonly present in fissured plaques, and that fissure frequently occurred at the junction of the fibrous cap with the adjacent normal endothelium. Using computer modelling for analysis of tensile stress across the vessel wall, these investigators found high concentrations of stress on the plaque cap overlying an area of lipid pool. In this area, the plaque cap lacks underlying collagen support which, perhaps, makes it more susceptible to rupture. Davies and co-workers suggested that the risk of fissuring can be predetermined by the plaque configuration and the biochemical and structural properties of the cap components [19,20].

Although the above experimental model is helpful in understanding the distribution of stress in plaques that protrude into the vessel lumen, it does not explain why rupture or ulceration occurs in plaques that are relatively flat and do not encroach into the lumen. A possible explanation for the latter process is that stress produced by turbulent flow in areas of stenosis or at branching points contributes to tearing of the plaque, particularly in the thinner portion of the fibrous cap. Therefore, not only intrinsic characteristics of the atherosclerotic lesion but forces external to the plaque itself, such as turbulence [26] or marked oscillation in shear stress [27] may contribute to the development of plaque growth and, perhaps, rupture. At this juncture, these are only speculations which require intensive investigations using animal experimentation and clinical observation.

Thrombus formation
The elegant work of Davies [1] and Falk [2] has clearly shown that thrombus forma-

tion secondary to atherosclerotic plaque disruption plays a fundamental role in the development of the acute coronary syndromes. Furthermore, emerging evidence suggests that this mechanism is also important in the progression of atherosclerosis even when symptoms are absent. In this section, we will discuss several evolving concepts pertaining to arterial thrombosis, including: (a) thrombus formation and organization; (b) labile versus fixed thrombus; (c) vasoconstriction, and (d) the effects of residual thrombi.

a) Thrombus formation and organization

Numerous pathologic studies on atherosclerotic plaques during the last decade [28,29] revealed the presence of old, organized coronary thrombi, which were difficult to distinguish from atherosclerotic changes seen in the arterial wall. According to these studies, organization of thrombi contributes to the progression to advanced atherosclerotic plaques. In the context of the most advanced atherosclerotic plaques, a more recent study by Falk [11] in patients with unstable angina leading to infarction or sudden death, revealed the presence of thrombi with layered appearance in the majority of cases. This suggested that recurrent episodes of mural thrombosis (rather than a single, abrupt thrombotic event) occurred, which eventually led to vascular occlusion [11]. Furthermore, the presence of small fragments of thrombotic material in the distal intramyocardial circulation suggested that intermittent thrombus formation and fragmentation commonly occurred. Further evidence supporting the role of thrombosis and thrombus incorporation in plaque progression is provided by a recent study by Bini et al. [30] using monoclonal antibody to identify fibrin, fibrinogen and fibrin(ogen) degradation products. They demonstrated that in advanced fibrous plaque, fibrin and fibrin-related products were detected in the intima, neointima, subintima, and even in the deeper medial layer, especially around thrombus, collagen and smooth muscle cells; on the other hand, fibrin and fibrin-related products were found in small quantities in early lesions and in normal arteries.

These thrombotic processes may or may not be associated with signs or symptoms of ischaemia. If mural thrombus formation does not result in significant reduction of myocardial perfusion, clinical evidence of ischaemia will probably be absent. On the other hand, partially or totally occlusive thrombi may lead to acute myocardial ischaemia or infarction (see below). Regardless of the presence or absence of symptoms, recurrent episodes of plaque disruption with superimposed thrombosis may lead to progressive narrowing of the coronary arteries. Indeed, in a study of 168 patients who underwent coronary angiography three times without undergoing coronary surgery or angioplasty, Bruschke et al. [31] demonstrated significant angiographic progression of coronary artery disease in a majority of patients who have no increase in cardiac symptoms. Although at present we do not know how prevalent this process of recurrent thrombosis is, it has potentially enormous clinical significance since thrombotic episodes may be prevented by platelet inhibitor or anticoagulant therapy. In this regard, the recently completed trial [32] of antiplatelet agents in the progression of atherosclerosis revealed that the use of aspirin and dipyridamole produced significant reduction in new lesion formation as assessed by angiography, and also a significant reduction in the incidence of myocardial infarction.

b) Labile versus fixed thrombus

Numerous angiographic reports [7,8,13-15,33-35] in the literature have documented the presence of intraluminal thrombi in both unstable angina and acute myocardial infarction. If plaque rupture and thrombosis are fundamental in the pathogenesis of acute ischaemic syndromes, why does one patient present with unstable angina and the other with myocardial infarction. This question was approached in the experimental laboratory using a perfusion chamber, in which different substrates were exposed to circulating blood at different shear rates [36]. When mild vascular injury was mimicked by exposing de-endothelialized aortic wall to circulating blood at different shear rates, platelet deposition reached maximum in 5 to 10 minutes. At higher shear rates and with longer exposure times, the thrombus was dislodged from the substrate by the flowing blood, suggesting that the thrombus was labile. On the other hand, when deep vessel injury was mimicked by using collagen type I as a substrate in the perfusion chamber [36], platelet deposition was markedly enhanced and the thrombus was not dislodged even at high shear rates.

In the clinical context, when injury to the vessel wall is mild, the thrombogenic stimulus may be relatively small and the resulting thrombotic occlusion transient, as occurs in unstable angina. Alternatively, deep vessel injury secondary to plaque rupture or ulceration results in exposure of collagen, lipids and other elements of the vessel media to the blood, leading to relatively persistent thrombotic occlusion and myocardial infarction [21]. Obviously, systemic factors (such as a hyperthrombotic state) and local factors (such as vasoconstriction, the presence of collaterals and myocardial oxygen demand) are important as well.

c) Vasoconstriction

Although a substantial proportion of episodes of unstable angina and acute myocardial infarction are caused by plaque fissuring or rupture with superimposed thrombosis, other mechanisms that alter the balance between myocardial oxygen supply and demand need to be considered. In this respect, studies by Maseri et al. [37], using haemodynamic and angiographic monitoring, have suggested that coronary vasospasm plays an important role in the pathogenesis of ischaemic heart disease. Indeed, vasospasm was found to be an important contributor to intermittent coronary occlusion in patients with acute myocardial infarction treated with intracoronary streptokinase, which responded, in some cases, to the administration of nitrates.

Several animal investigations aimed at elucidating the pathophysiology of vasoconstriction in coronary disease have been published recently. In the porcine model of carotid angioplasty [38], vasoconstriction proximal and distal to the angioplasty site was observed, which was proportional to the degree of platelet deposition and lasted for about 5-15 minutes. Furthermore, vasoconstriction was partially inhibited by pretreatment with aspirin, suggesting that the interaction of platelets with the vessel wall and the subsequent release of vasoactive substances are important in the development of vasospasm.

In a different set of experiments using a canine preparation of severe coronary artery stenosis, Folts et al. [39] demonstrated the presence of cyclic variations in coronary flow, which were presumed to be caused by platelet aggregation at the stenotic site. Subsequent study by Ashton et al. [40] demonstrated that serotonin and thromboxane A2 were important mediators of the cyclic flow variations, and that pharmacologic blockade of these substances frequently abolished them.

There is additional evidence suggesting that atherosclerotic arteries have an abnormal vascular tone, perhaps related to a deficiency in the production or release of endothelium-derived relaxing factor [41]. Indeed, when the vasodilator acetylcholine was administered into the coronary arteries of patients with early and advanced atherosclerosis, vasoconstriction was observed [42]. Furthermore, animal experiments have shown that damaged endothelium responds abnormally to vasoactive substances such as acetylcholine and bradykinin [43] and that vessels with even early atherosclerosis have increased vasoconstrictor response to serotonin and thromboxane A2, as well as impaired vasodilator response to adenosine diphosphate [44]. Based on these data, it appears that atherosclerosis is associated with an exaggerated vasoconstrictor response triggered by humoral factors and is secondary to the loss of the endothelium-derived relaxing factor, which may be important in the pathogenesis of circadian coronary vasospasm in patients with acute ischaemic syndromes.

d) Residual thrombus: increased thrombogenicity

Spontaneous lysis of thrombus appears to play a role not only in unstable angina but also in acute myocardial infarction. In these patients, as well as in those undergoing thrombolysis for acute infarction, the presence of a residual mural thrombus predisposes to recurrent thrombotic vessel occlusion. Two main contributing factors for the development of rethrombosis have been identified.

First, the residual mural thrombus may encroach into the vessel lumen, resulting in an increased shear rate which facilitates the activation and deposition of platelets on the lesion. In this context, using an experimental animal model of ex-vivo perfusion, Badimon et al. [45] have shown that platelet deposition is higher with increasing degrees of vessel stenosis. This is probably due to the fact that luminal stenosis alters the laminar flow, increases the shear rate and facilitates the interaction of platelets with the vessel wall.

Second, the presence of a residual thrombus is one of the most powerful thrombogenic surfaces ever encountered in the laboratory [46]. This was also evaluated in an ex-vivo perfusion model, where platelet deposition was assessed by continuous scintigraphic imaging of indium-111-labelled platelets. A gradual increase in platelet deposition in the area of maximal stenosis was observed, followed by an abrupt drop, probably due to spontaneous thrombus embolization or platelet disaggregation. This was immediately followed by a rapid increase in platelet deposition, suggesting that the remaining thrombus was markedly thrombogenic [21,46].

The results of the aforementioned experiments can be interpreted in the light of clinical data in patients with acute myocardial infarction undergoing thrombolysis, which has shown that residual vessel stenosis [47,48] and intracoronary thrombus [48,49] were associated with an increased risk of thrombotic reocclusion. Further research into the mechanisms of platelet and clotting activation during thrombolysis, and measures to prevent reocclusion, is currently underway.

Pathophysiology of acute ischaemic syndromes

Using the above concepts regarding plaque rupture and thrombosis as a framework, we will discuss the pathophysiology of the acute coronary syndromes (Table 2).

Table 2. Pathogenesis of the acute ischaemic syndromes.

Syndrome	Substrate damage	Thrombus	
		Fixed	Labile
Unstable angina(#)	+	+	+++
Non-Q-wave infarction(#,*)	++	++	++
Q-wave infarction(#,*)	+++	+++	+

+ = Mild; ++ = Moderate; +++ = Severe
# Vasoconstriction may contribute to coronary occlusion
* Collaterals may decrease the extension of infarction
Note: In sudden ischaemic death, substrate damage ranges from mild to severe; absence of collaterals or presence of platelet microemboli may be contributory factors.

In unstable angina, a relatively small fissuring or disruption at an atherosclerotic plaque may lead to an acute change in plaque morphology and a reduction in coronary blood flow, resulting in exacerbation of angina. Transient episodes of thrombotic vessel occlusion at the site of plaque injury may occur, leading to angina at rest [9]. This thrombus is usually labile, and results in temporary vessel occlusion, perhaps lasting only 10-20 minutes [21,35]. In addition, release of vasoactive substances by platelets and vasoconstriction secondary to endothelial vasodilator dysfunction may contribute to a reduction in coronary flow. Alterations in perfusion and myocardial oxygen supply probably account for two-thirds of patients with unstable angina; the rest may be caused by transient increases in myocardial oxygen demand. Indeed, in a study by Langer *et al.* [50] in 196 patients with unstable angina, they demonstrated, with the use of Holter-ST segment analysis, that an increase in rate-pressure product precedes the onset of ST segment shift in 75% of episodes. They concluded that myocardial ischaemia in patients with unstable angina may be mediated in part by an increased myocardial oxygen demand.

In non-Q-wave infarction, the angiographic morphology of the responsible lesion is similar to that seen in unstable angina, suggesting that plaque disruption is common to both syndromes [8]. About one-quarter of patients with non-Q-wave infarction have a completely occluded infarct-related vessel at early angiography, with the distal territory usually supplied by collaterals [34]. In the remaining patients, the infarct-related artery is patent. The presence of ST segment elevation in the electrocardiogram, an early peak in plasma creatine kinase, and a high angiographic patency rate of the involved vessel, suggest that complete coronary occlusion followed by early reperfusion (within the first two hours) or resolution of vasospasm are pathogenetically important in non-Q-wave infarction [51,52]. We speculate that in this syndrome, plaque damage is of greater severity than in unstable angina, resulting in relatively more persistent thrombotic occlusion. Spontaneous thrombolysis or spasm resolution, however, limit the duration of myocardial ischaemia and prevent the formation of Q-wave infarction.

In Q-wave infarction, plaque rupture may be associated with deep arterial injury or ulceration, resulting in the formation of a fixed and persistent thrombus. These lead to an abrupt cessation of myocardial perfusion and, eventually, to necrosis of the involved myocardium. The coronary lesion responsible for the infarction is frequently only mildly to moderately stenotic [14-17], which suggests that plaque rupture with superimposed thrombosis is the primary determinant of acute occlusion, rather than the severity of the underlying lesion [14-17]. It is conceivable that in patients with severe coronary stenosis, well-developed collaterals prevent or reduce the extent of infarction [21,53]. In perhaps one-quarter of patients, coronary thrombosis results from superficial intimal injury or blood stasis in areas of high-grade stenosis [19]; such a mechanism has been reproduced in the experimental model [39,45]. Additionally, myocardial infarction may be promoted by alterations in haemostasis, such as increased activation of the coagulation system, increased platelet aggregability, elevated fibrinogen and Factor VII activity, or deficient fibrinolytic mechanisms.

Finally, sudden coronary death probably involves a rapidly progressive coronary lesion, in which plaque rupture and resultant thrombosis [1,2,11] lead to ischaemia and fatal ventricular arrthymias. The absence of collateral flow to the myocardium distal to the occlusion or platelet microemboli [11], perhaps contributes to the development of sudden ischaemic death.

Future antithrombotic approach

The effectiveness of aspirin has been unequivocally demonstrated in acute ischaemic syndromes as well as in clinical conditions in which the thrombotic risk is high, such as in patients receiving vein graft bypass and coronary angioplasty [21,46,54,55]. It is of interest that aspirin only interferes with one of the three pathways of platelet activation; the other two pathways (dependent on adenosine diphosphate and collagen and thrombin) remain unaffected. It is not surprising, therefore, that aspirin cannot completely prevent platelet-related thrombotic events. Several other emerging antithrombotic modalities in the management of the acute ischaemic syndromes will be discussed below.

a) Combination therapy

Combination therapy with low dose aspirin and an anticoagulant may prove effective in patients at high risk for thrombotic events, such as those with unstable angina, acute myocardial infarction, and following coronary thrombolysis or revascularization. The rationale behind this combination is to block one of the pathways of platelet activation and also the generation of thrombin by the intrinsic and extrinsic coagulation systems. Thrombin itself is not only a powerful platelet activator but it also leads to the formation and crosslinking of fibrin, which in turn provides stabilization to the growing platelet thrombus (Fig. 1).

b) Thrombin inhibitors

Hirudin is a potent and specific thrombin inhibitor, initially isolated from the salivary glands of the medicinal leech but recently synthesized by recombinant DNA

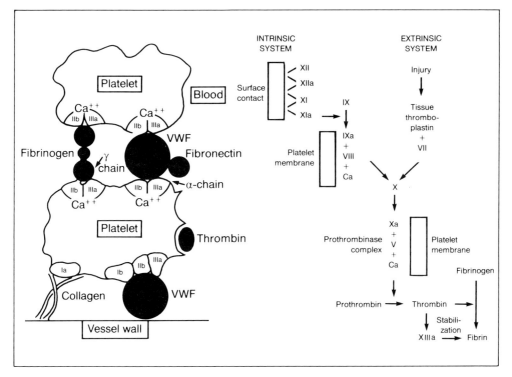

Fig. 1. The role of platelets and the coagulation system in the pathogenesis of thrombus formation following vascular injury. The mechanisms in platelet aggregation and activation of coagulation factors following vascular injury are illustrated here.

techniques. Hirudin prevents activation of coagulation factors V, VIII and XIII; in addition, being a powerful inhibitor of thrombin formation, it prevents platelet aggregation induced by this enzyme. Hirudin has recently been shown to prevent thrombosis in an animal model of carotid angioplasty [56]. Other peptide inhibitors of thrombin have been synthesized and tested in animal models [57]. A synthetic covalent inhibitor of thrombin was found to effectively inhibit platelet haemostatic plug formation and vascular graft thrombosis [57]. The potential clinical utilities of these agents in the management of the acute ischaemic syndromes awaits further experimental and clinical testing.

c) Receptor blockers

Intense investigation has been focused on the development of monoclonal antibodies against platelet membrane receptors and adhesive macromolecules. Thus far, the results from in-vitro animal studies have been encouraging. A monoclonal antibody against von Willebrand factor was found to be significantly more potent than aspirin in terms of platelet thrombus inhibition in an ex-vivo perfusion animal model [58]. Another monoclonal antibody directed against the platelet receptor glycoprotein receptor IIb-IIIa, reduced platelet thrombus formation on artificial vascular graft and enhanced thrombolysis when added to tissue plasminogen activator in an experimental model of coronary thrombosis [59].

References

[1] Davies MJ, Thomas AC.
Plaque fissuring — the cause of acute myocardial infarction, sudden ischaemic death, and crescendo angina.
Br Heart J 1985; **53**: 363–73.

[2] Falk E.
Plaque rupture with severe pre-existing stenosis precipitating coronary thrombosis. Characteristics of coronary atherosclerotic plaques underlying fatal occlusive thrombi.
Br Heart J 1983; **50**: 127–34.

[3] Benson RL.
The present status of coronary arterial disease.
Arch Pathol 1926; **2**: 870–916.

[4] Constantinides P.
Plaque fissuring in human coronary thrombosis.
J Atheroscler Res 1966; **6**: 1–17.

[5] Chandler AB.
Mechanism and frequency of thrombosis in the coronary circulation.
Thromb Res 1974; **4**: 3–22.

[6] Fulton WFM.
The coronary arteries. Arteriography, microanatomy and pathogenesis of obliterative coronary disease.
Springfield: Charles C. Thomas, 1986; 230–96.

[7] Ambrose JA, Winters SL, Stern A, et al.
Angiographic morphology and the pathogenesis of unstable angina pectoris.
J Am Coll Cardiol 1985; **5**: 609–16.

[8] Ambrose JA, Hjemdale-Monsen CE, Borrico S, Gorlin R, Fuster V.
Angiographic demonstration of a common link between unstable angina pectoris and non-Q wave acute myocardial infarction.
Am J Cardiol 1988; **61**: 244–7.

[9] Sherman CT, Litvak F, Grundfest W, et al.
Coronary angioscopy in patients with unstable angina pectoris.
N Engl J Med 1986; **315**: 913–9.

[10] Levin DC, Fallon JT.
Significance of the angiographic morphology of localized coronary stenosis: histopathologic correlations.
Circulation 1982; **66**: 316–20.

[11] Falk E.
Unstable angina with fatal outcome: dynamic coronary thrombosis leading to infarction and/or sudden death. Autopsy evidence of recurrent mural thrombosis with peripheral embolization culminating in total vascular occlusion.
Circulation 1985; **71**: 699–708.

[12] Moise A, Lesperance J, Theroux P, et al.
Clinical and angiographic predictors of new total coronary occlusion in coronary artery disease. Analysis of 313 nonoperated patients.
Am J Cardiol 1984; **54**: 1176–81.

[13] Ambrose JA, Winters SL, Arora RR, et al.
Angiographic evolution of coronary artery morphology in unstable angina.
J Am Coll Cardiol 1986; **7**: 472–8.

[14] Ambrose JA, Tannenbaum M, Alexoupolous D, et al.
Angiographic progression of coronary artery disease and the development of myocardial infarction.
J Am Coll Cardiol 1988; **12**: 56–62.

[15] Little WC, Constantinescui M, Applegate RT.
Can coronary angiography predict the site of a subsequent myocardial infarction in patients with mild to moderate coronary artery disease.
Circulation 1988; **78**: 457–66.

[16] Brown GB, Gallery CA, Badger RS, et al.
Incomplete lysis of thrombus in the moderate underlying atherosclerotic lesion during intracoronary infusion of streptokinase for acute myocardial infarction:Quantitative angiographic observations.
Circulation 1986; **73**: 653–61.

[17] McPherson DD, Hiratzka LF, Lamberth WC, et al.
Delineation of the extent of coronary atherosclerosis by high frequency epicardial echocardiography.
N Engl J Med 1987; **316**: 304–9.

[18] Glagov S, Weisenberg E, Zarins CK, Stantunavicius R, Kolettis GJ.
Compensatory enlargement of atherosclerotic human coronary arteries.
N Engl J Med 1987; **316**: 1371–5.

[19] Davies MJ.
Thrombosis and coronary atherosclerosis.
In: Julian DG, Kubler W, Norris RM, Swan HJ, Collen D, Verstrate M, eds. *Thrombolysis in Cardiovascular Disease.* New York: Marcel Dekker, 1989; 25–43.

[20] Richardson PD, Davies MJ, Born GV.
Influence of plaque configuration and stress distribution in fissuring of coronary atherosclerotic plaque.
Lancet 1989; **i**: 941–4.

[21] Fuster V, Badimon L, Cohen M, Ambrose JA, Badimon JJ, Chesebro JH.
Insights into the pathogenesis of acute ischemic syndromes.
Circulation 1988; **77**: 1213–20.

[22] Fuster V, Bowie JW, Lewis JC, et al.
Resistance to atherosclerosis in pigs with von Willebrand disease. Spontaneous and high cholesterol diet-induced arteriosclerosis.
J Clin Invest 1978; **61**: 722–30.

[23] Fuster V, Fass DN, Kaye MP, et al.
Arteriosclerosis in normal and von Willebrand pigs. Long term prospective study and aortic transplantation.
Circ Res 1982; **51**: 587–93.

[24] Ross R.
The pathogenesis of atherosclerosis — an update.
N Engl J Med 1986; **314**: 488–500.

[25] Mitchinson MJ, Ball RY.
Macrophages and atherosclerosis.
Lancet 1987; **ii**: 146–9.

[26] Weinberger J, Ramos L, Ambrose JA, Fuster V.
Morphologic and dynamic changes of atherosclerotic plaque at the carotid artery bifurcation: sequential imaging by real time B-mode ultrasonography.
J Am Coll Cardiol 1988; **12**: 1515–21.

[27] Ku DN, Giddens DP, Zarins CK, Glagov S.
Pulsatile flow and atherosclerosis in the human carotid bifurcation. Positive correlation between plaque location and low and oscillatory shear stress.
Arteriosclerosis 1985; **5**: 293–302.

[28] Roberts WC, Buja LM.
The frequency and significance of coronary arterial thrombi and other observations in fatal acute myocardial infarction. A study of 107 patients.
Am J Med 1972; **52**: 425–43.

[29] Ridolfi RL, Hutchins GM.
The relationship between coronary artery lesions and myocardial infarcts. Ulceration of atherosclerotic plaques precipitating coronary thrombosis.
Am Heart J 1977; **93**: 468–86.

[30] Bini A, Fanoglio JJ, Mesa-Tejada R, Kudryk B, Kaplan KL.
Identification and distribution of fibrinogen, fibrin, and fibrin(ogen) degradation products in atherosclerosis. Use of monoclonal antibodies.
Arteriosclerosis 1989; **9**: 109–21.

[31] Bruschke AVG, Kramer JR, Bal ET, et al.
The dynamics of progression of coronary atherosclerosis studied in 168 medically treated patients who underwent coronary arteriography three times.
Am Heart J 1989; **117**: 296–305.

[32] Chesebro JH, Webster MW, Smith HC, et al.
Antiplatelet therapy in coronary artery disease progression: reduced infarction and new lesion formation. [Abstract]
Circulation 1989; **80** (suppl. II):II–266.

[33] DeWood MA, Spores J, Notske R, et al.
Prevalence of total coronary occlusion during the early hours of transluminal myocardial infarction.
N Engl J Med 1980; **303**: 897–902.

[34] DeWood MA, Stifter WF, Simpson CS, et al.
Coronary arteriographic findings soon after non-Q wave myocardial infarction.
N Engl J Med 1986; **315**: 417–23.

[35] Gotoh K, Minamino P, Haton O, *et al.*
The role of intracoronary thrombus in
unstable angina: angiographic assessment
and thrombolytic therapy during ongoing
anginal attacks.
Circulation 1988; **77**: 526–34.

[36] Badimon L, Badimon JJ, Galvez A,
Chesebro JH, Fuster V.
Influence of arterial damage and wall shear
rate on platelet deposition. Ex vivo study in
a swine model.
Arteriosclerosis 1986; **6**: 312–20.

[37] Maseri A, L'Abbate A, Chierchia S, *et al.*
Significance of spasm in the pathogenesis of
ischemic heart disease.
Am J Cardiol 1979; **44**: 788–92.

[38] Lam JYT, Chesebro JH, Steele PM,
Badimon L, Fuster V.
Is vasospasm related to platelet deposition?
Relationship in a porcine preparation of
arterial injury in vivo.
Circulation 1987; **75**: 243–8.

[39] Folts JD, Gallagher K, Rowe GG.
Blood flow reductions in stenosed canine
coronary arteries: vasospasm or platelet
aggregation?
Circulation 1982; **65**: 248–55.

[40] Ashton JH, Benedict CR, Fitzgerald C, *et al.*
Serotonin as a mediator of cyclic flow
variations in stenosed canine coronary
arteries.
Circulation 1986; **73**: 572–8.

[41] Griffith TM, Lewis MJ, Newby AC,
Henderson AH.
Endothelium-derived relaxing factor.
J Am Coll Cardiol 1988; **12**: 797–805.

[42] Ludmer PL, Selwyn AP, Shook TL, *et al.*
Paradoxical vasoconstriction induced by
acetylcholine in atherosclerotic coronary
arteries.
N Engl J Med 1986; **315**: 1046–51.

[43] Penny WJ, Chesebro JH, Heras M, Badimon
L, Fuster V.
In vivo identification of normal and
damaged endothelium by quantitative
coronary angiography and infusion of
acetylcholine and bradykinin in pigs.
[Abstract]
J Am Coll Cardiol 1988; **11** (suppl. A): 29A.

[44] Lopez JAG, Armstrong ML, Piegors DJ,
Heistad DD.
Effect of early and advanced atherosclerosis
on vascular responses to serotonin,
thromboxane A2 and ADP.
Circulation 1989; **79**: 698–705.

[45] Badimon L, Badimon JJ, Turitto VT,
Chesebro JH, Fuster V.
Mechanisms of arterial thrombosis: platelet
thrombus formation in areas of stenosis.
[Abstract]
Circulation 1987; **76** (suppl. IV): IV–102.

[46] Fuster V, Stein B, Badimon L, Chesebro JH.
Antithrombotic therapy after myocardial
reperfusion in acute myocardial infarction.
J Am Coll Cardiol 1988; **12** (suppl. A): 78A–
84A.

[47] Badger RS, Brown BG, Kennedy JW, *et al.*
Usefulness of recanalization of luminal
diameter of 0.6 millimeters or more with
intracoronary streptokinase during acute
myocardial infarction in predicting normal
perfusion status, continued arterial patency
and survival at one year.
Am J Cardiol 1987; **59**: 519–22.

[48] Harrison DG, Ferguson DW, Collins SM, *et
al.*
Rethrombosis after reperfusion with
streptokinase: importance of geometry of
residual lesions.
Circulation 1984; **69**: 991–9.

[49] De Guise P, Theroux P, Bonan R, Levy G,
Crepeau J.
Rethrombosis after successful thrombolysis
and angioplasty in acute myocardial
infarction.
J Am Coll Cardiol 1988; **11** (suppl. A): 192A.

[50] Langer A, Freeman M, Armstrong PW.
ST segment shift in unstable angina:
pathophysiology and association with
coronary anatomy and hospital outcome.
J Am Coll Cardiol 1989; **13**: 1495–1502.

[51] Gibson RS, Beller GA, Gheorghiade M, *et
al.*
The prevalence and clinical significance of
residual myocardial ischemia 2 weeks after
uncomplicated non-Q wave infarction. A
prospective natural history study.
Circulation 1986; **73**: 1186–98.

[52] Timmis AD, Griffin B, Grick JCP, Nelson
DJ, Sowton E.
The effects of early coronary patency on the
evolution of myocardial infarction: a
prospective arteriographic study.
Br Heart J 1987; **58**: 345–51.

[53] Rentrop PK, Feit F, Thornton JC.
The protective potential of collaterals
depends on the time of their development.
[Abstract]
J Am Coll Cardiol 1990; **15**: 202A.

[54] Resnekov L, Chediak J, Hirsch J, Lewis D.
Antithrombotic agents in coronary artery
disease.
Chest 1989; **95** (suppl.): 52S–72S.

[55] Fuster V, Chesebro JH.
Role of platelets and platelet inhibitors in
aortocoronary artery vein-graft disease.
Circulation 1986; **73**: 227–32.

[56] Heras M, Chesebro JH, Penny WJ, Bailey KR, Badimon L, Fuster V.
Effects of thrombin inhibitor on the development of acute platelet-thrombus deposition during angioplasty in pigs. Heparin versus recombinant hirudin, a specific thrombin inhibitor.
Circulation 1989; **79:** 657–65.

[57] Hanson SR, Harker LA.
Interruption of acute platelet-dependent thrombosis by the synthetic antithrombin D-phenylalanyl-L-prolyl-L-arginyl choromethy ketone.
Proc Natl Acad Sci USA 1988; **85:** 3184–8.

[58] Hanson SR, Pareti FI, Ruggeri ZM, *et al.*
Effects of monoclonal antibody against the platelet glycoprotein IIb/IIIa complex on thrombosis and hemostasis in the baboon.
J Clin Invest 1988; **81:** 149–58.

[59] Gold HK, Coller BS, Yasuda T, *et al.*
Rapid and sustained coronary artery recanalization with combined bolus injection of recombination tissue-type plasminogen activator and monoclonal antiplatelet GPIIb/IIIa antibody in a canine preparation.
Circulation 1988; **77:** 670–77.

CORONARY ANGIOSCOPY AND MYOCARDIAL ISCHAEMIA

J.S. FORRESTER

At the Cedars-Sinai Medical Center, the nature of the coronary endothelial surface on angioscopic examination has been shown to determine clinical outcome: stable angina; accelerated angina; rest angina, and myocardial infarction.

Stable angina

Fig. 1 shows a coronary angiogram in a patient with stable angina; this lesion was graded by angiographers as a 75% stenosis. What would that lesion look like if it were

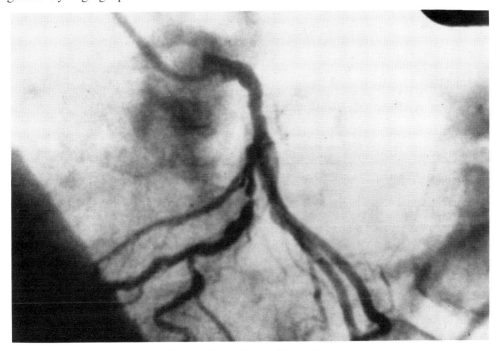

Fig. 1. Coronary angiogram in a patient with stable angina.

to be viewed from within? Fig. 2 gives the cine image of that lesion as seen by angioscopy; the atheroma producing about a 70% stenosis can be seen, with a smooth surface without evidence of endothelial disruption.

Ideas on the pathogenesis of myocardial infarction relate back many years. Meyer Friedman did some superb pathologic work in the 1960s, and Fig. 3 presents one of his slides. A fibrous cap lying over an Oil-Red O stained mass of lipid can be seen, with a necrotic core. This necrotic core is frequently lined by macrophages and it is my belief, based on the work of pathology colleagues, that it is erosion of this necrotic core upwards through the fibrous cap that initiates the phenomenon of fibrous cap disruption leading to thrombus formation.

At the Cedars-Sinai Medical Center we have data to support this proposition from studies using monoclonal antibodies to detect two cytokines produced by macrophages — tumour necrosis factor and interleukin 1. These cytokines have some interesting properties. First, they are cytotoxic to certain cells; second, they are among the most powerful of the cytokines to produce neovascularization, which is typical of atheroma progression; third, they may have some potential role in evolution of the plaque. We have found that as the plaque progresses from normal vessel — where there is no tumour necrosis factor or interleukin 1 — to plaque disruption, there is a

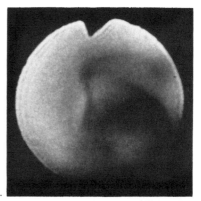

Fig. 2. Angioscopic image of the lesion seen in Fig. 1.

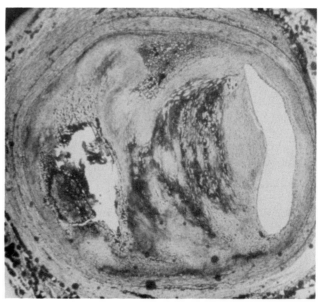

Fig. 3. Pathologic appearance of a fibrous plaque. (Reproduced with permission from Friedman M, *Am J Pathol* 1965; **48:** 19.)

substantial increase in the frequency of macrophage positivity for these two compounds. So I believe that there is emerging evidence that the macrophage produces compounds that are capable of causing plaque evolution and, ultimately, plaque disruption.

Accelerated angina

Stable angina can progress to accelerated angina. Fig. 4 shows an angioscopic image of a lesion that by angiography was very similar to Fig. 1. Although the angiographic image was similar, by angioscopy it looks very different. There is haemorrhage and, proceeding down the vessel, there is torn endothelium protruding into the intervascular space — very different from the smooth surface endothelium in Fig. 1. While the tear may seem slight, it is enough, I believe, to cause the syndrome of accelerated angina. There is a necrotic core and an erosion of the fibrous cap with tearing of the endothelial surface.

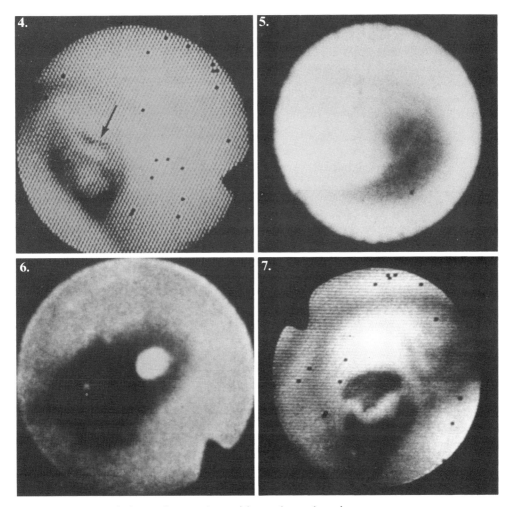

Fig. 4.   Angioscopic image in a patient with accelerated angina.

Fig. 5.   Angioscopic image in a patient with unstable rest angina.

Fig. 6.   Angioscopic image in a patient with developing myocardial infarction.

Fig. 7.   Angioscopic image of intimal tearing after balloon angioplasty.

In the last year, we have accumulated data regarding the unstable atherosclerotic plaque. The region surrounding the area of endothelial disruption was found to have a substantial increase in frequency of mast cells. Further, an increase in the number of mast cell granules and the frequency of degranulation was shown in lesions that have intimal disruption. Hence, I believe that we have evidence, from immunohistochemistry and from the frequency and distribution of mast cells, for atheroma progression.

Rest angina

Angioscopy of unstable rest angina (distinguished from accelerated angina by the additional component of instability with rest pain) is presented as Fig. 5. There is a crescent-shaped, partially occlusive thrombus in an individual about to have a myocardial infarction.

A comparison of the three syndromes discussed thus far shows variation in the frequency of intimal damage and thrombus formation in each. A great majority of patients with stable angina have smooth plaque; in 5% of patients there is intimal damage and ulceration without acute syndrome. In accelerated angina the great majority of patients have intimal ulceration, but there are also patients who have no clear evidence of intimal ulceration. In unstable rest angina — very severe chest pain syndrome — a partially occlusive thrombus was found in 12 out of 13 cases. Thus, the conclusion may be drawn that acute coronary syndromes are primarily caused by intimal ulceration and thrombus. It should be noted that the patients reviewed here are those referred for bypass surgery, and it may be that such patients show a much higher frequency of intimal disruption and thrombus than less seriously ill individuals.

Fig. 6 shows an angioscopic image from a patient with developing myocardial infarction. There is a totally occlusive thrombus with haemorrhage radiating out from it, and some torn endothelium around the periphery. Nine days prior he had had a partially occlusive thrombus detected by angiography. This supports the idea of thrombus progression over time. The thrombus need not, but it can, evolve episodically, hence leaving a window of opportunity for preventive therapy.

Myocardial infarction

Angioscopic images at various stages following myocardial infarction show a typical progression. One day following myocardial infarction, we have found partially occlusive thrombus despite the absence of any thrombolytic therapy. At one week post-myocardial infarction, we have found that the thrombus has been cleaned up; but there is often a torn and irregular intimal surface, suggesting that thrombus formation is involved in myocardial infarction and that thrombolysis can occur spontaneously. At two months following myocardial infarction, we have found haemorrhage and, notably, strands of torn endothelium. I believe that such tears have major potential as sites of platelet aggregation and dislodgement, in keeping with the work of Dr Michael Davies and others who have shown the presence of emboli distal to the site of current or prior thrombus formation.

The potential significance of intimal tearing is apparent in Fig. 7. This is an image of iatrogenically-induced acute coronary syndrome after angiographically successful balloon angioplasty. The intimal surface is terribly torn; there is a double lumen created by the angioplaster and severe haemorrhage. The 'successful' angioplasty failed at 48 hours, leading to bypass surgery. So the potential for balloon angioplasty to produce, in effect, the same endothelial damage that occurs biologically must be borne in mind.

Excimer laser angioplasty

A new approach to the problem of recanalization of an artery is excimer laser angioplasty. Fig. 8 is an angiogram from a patient who had a saphenous vein bypass graft and who had cardiac arrest outside the hospital. There is a very severe stenosis in the bypass graft leading to the right coronary artery. This 85-year-old lady had previously undergone bypass surgery and three balloon angioplasties at this location with re-stenosis. The other three panels of the figure illustrate that same blood vessel following placement of the excimer laser catheter, laser angioplasty and follow up balloon angioplasty. By passing a catheter down through the graft, bringing the excimer laser catheter directly up to the stenosis and then slowly passing it through, vessel patency was restored in a matter of a minute or so. The great potential of this technique is that we believe it vaporizes the plaque, as opposed to balloon angioplasty which simply presses it up against the wall. The excimer laser should also be useful in a situation of diffuse disease in which balloon angioplasty would not be particularly applicable.

The excimer laser is of great potential interest in cardiology. It has very high power and can vaporize virtually any kind of obstruction, yet it is very superficial in its cutting so it does not produce any lateral burn injury. This allows blood vessels to be opened up without producing spasm. It may therefore be possible in the future to prevent the development of acute coronary syndromes simply by vaporizing and entirely

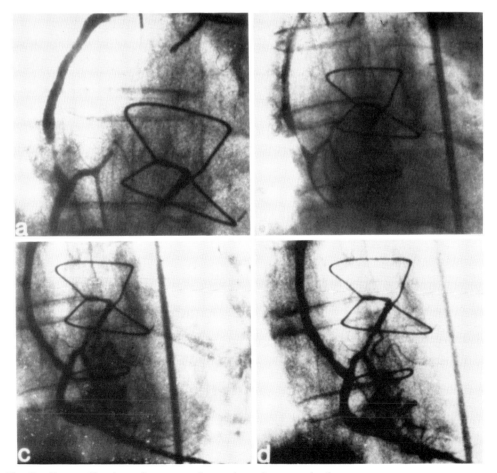

Fig. 8. Recanalization of an artery by excimer laser angioplasty.

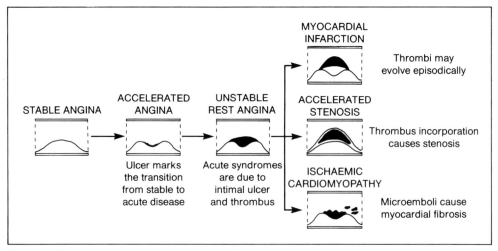

Fig. 9. The ulceration-thrombosis cycle of coronary disease.

removing the obstructions. Within the next ten years I believe it will be possible to re-store the vessel to its original diameter and solve the problem of re-stenosis.

Conclusion

We should endeavour to relate clinical syndromes to intimal pathology and, of course, the intimal pathology seen at angioscopy to that demonstrated by histologic studies. Results of these different studies are compatible with an ulceration-thrombosis cycle of coronary disease (Fig. 9). I believe that stable angina is due to stable atheroma. When the stable atheroma becomes unstable and ulcerates it produces accelerated angina. In a majority of cases, the patient with accelerated angina may go on to heal; with ulcer healing, however, there is stenosis progression. The ulceration may also develop to become a partially occlusive thrombus, producing the more severe syn-drome of unstable rest angina. In turn, the partially occlusive thrombus may be incor-porated, again with stenosis progression, or it may become a larger, partially occlusive thrombus. Intimal ulceration can also lead to platelet aggregation and dislodgement; I believe that dislodgement of the platelets and thrombus that form on the intimal ulceration is an important mechanism of sudden death in some patients. So, in effect, there are two cycles, an ulceration cycle and a thrombus cycle. These may give rise to a 'punctuated equilibrium' in which long periods of stability are punctuated by sudden episodes of plaque disruption that return, ultimately, to stability.

References

[1] Forrester JS, Litvack F, Grundfest W, Fishbein M.
A perspective of coronary disease seen through the arteries of living man.
Circulation 1987; **75**: 505–13.

[2] Sherman CT, Litvack F, Grundfest W, *et al.*
Demonstration of thrombus and complex atheroma by in-vivo angioscopy in patients with unstable angina pectoris.
N Engl J Med 1986; **315**: 913–9.

CORONARY VASOMOTION IN ACUTE ISCHAEMIA

A. MASERI, G. DAVIES

How prevalent is vasomotion/vasospasm in the context of acute coronary occlusion? The most obvious finding in studies of coronary occlusion is a red thrombus, the type Dr Falk (see page 1) describes as a venous clot. Such a clot is both the consequence of occlusion and the cause of its persistence and extension, but as such it represents a relatively late development. The initial formation of a red thrombus depends on the local balance between thrombosis/thrombolysis, blood platelets, and spasm or constriction, because persistent occlusion is a prerequisite for the development of red thrombus. Such occlusion may result from the formation of a white thrombus, arising from the gradual deposition of platelets from flowing blood. Alternatively, if there is responsive smooth muscle in the artery wall, spasm or constriction may occur and this can produce persistent occlusion.

Pathophysiology of coronary occlusion

The question then is what prompts initial occlusion of a coronary vessel. It may be convenient to attribute this to plaque fissuring, which is after all a most conspicuous event, but the process may well be much more complex. When unstable angina and the early stages of myocardial infarction are analysed it is apparent that these phenomena display 'stuttering evolution', with thrombus forming and breaking down repeatedly so that thrombi of different ages are seen. If tremendous thrombogenic potential was present, it would be expected to precipitate catastrophic thrombus formation, as seen with the introduction of thrombogenic prostheses in animals. The fact that this does not occur in many cases in which the occlusion is initially occasional and then intermittent suggests that the thrombogenic potential is not so great. This may be due to properties of the vessel wall that render it less thrombogenic or enhance fibrinolysis, or to a diminished response of the blood to thrombogenic stimuli. Alternatively, it may be due to changes in blood flow; stagnation at a site of vessel constriction might initiate the growth of a red thrombus.

The role of vasospasm

What evidence exists implicating vasospasm with coronary occlusion? A few years ago, David Hackett and colleagues studied this issue in 45 patients with early acute myocardial infarction. Patients received intracoronary isosorbide dinitrate (2-4 mg), followed by thrombolytic therapy (up to 600,000 IU streptokinase) [1]. In those patients who at the very end of thrombolysis had severe residual stenosis with poor run off, a further 2 mg bolus of intracoronary nitrate restored full patency in 11 of 16 patients. These are results strongly supportive of a vasoconstrictor component in at least some patients with acute coronary occlusion.

Another feature of these results was the variable extent of stenosis after thrombolysis. Hackett *et al.* [2] examined this in a group of 60 patients presenting with first myocardial infarction. This data reveals two interesting facts. The first is the wide variation in degree of stenosis — in at least 20% of these patients stenosis is not very severe, a result congruent with the TAMI II trial in which 12.6% of patients had post-thrombolysis stenoses too small to permit randomization to angioplasty. The second point is that thrombolysis may not remove all the thrombotic material present. In 40 out of 48 patients in whom recanalization of vessels was achieved, the size of the infarct-related stenosis was further reduced by isosorbide dinitrate.

In parallel with this, workers in the Cardiovascular Unit at the Royal Postgraduate Medical School, Hammersmith Hospital, have undertaken studies in collaboration with Margarita Vejar and Carlo Patrono. Urinary thromboxane B_2 was measured in patients receiving isosorbide and diltiazem for unstable angina and was correlated with ischaemic ST-segment changes recorded during continuous electrocardiogram (ECG) monitoring to determine if variations in urinary thromboxane correspond to episodes of silent ischaemia [3,4]. This appears not to be the case, a result which suggests that thrombotic processes may go on without causing complete obstruction. Another interesting feature of this work is that some subjects were receiving aspirin at doses that should virtually abolish thromboxane production by platelets, yet in some of these subjects quite remarkable increases in urinary thromboxane levels were apparent. This may be due to incomplete blockade of platelet thromboxane synthesis; equally, however, it may be an indication that there are thromboxane-synthesizing cells in the vessel wall.

Vasoconstriction and vasospasm

A clear distinction should be drawn between vasoconstriction and occlusive vasospasm. Variant angina is a good example of vasospasm and David Hackett's [5] investigations into this phenomenon have produced results which help to outline the quantitative differences between spasm and constriction. Following intracoronary ergonovine, spastic artery segments in affected patients show complete occlusion whereas in the non-spastic segments in the same patient only a mild constriction occurs reducing the calibre by about 10%-20%, very similar to the response of vessels in subjects who do not have angina. This observation indicates the presence of a segmental coronary artery hyperreactivity which results in local occlusion in response to stimuli which cause only mild constriction in adjacent segments. Juan Carlos Kaski found that this was the case also during spontaneous spasm [6,7].

Complementary findings have been reported by Ben Freedman and his colleagues [8]. In their study, the geometric theory of MacAlpin was used to predict the degree of constriction likely to result from ergonovine challenge, on the basis of the degree of existing stenosis. It is interesting to observe that while actual responses to ergonovine in patients with variant angina were consistently greater than predicted, responses in the control group were almost always less than expected. The essence of spasm, then, is an enhanced responsiveness to stimuli in susceptible vessel segments [6]. In the case of variant angina, it would seem that this hyperreactivity is inherent in the vessel segments and is not dependent on the stimulant used — ergonovine, dopamine, histamine, cold-pressor stress or hand-grip challenge all of which induce a similar response although acting through different receptor mechanisms, and that response is always complete obstruction rather than just mild change [9].

These findings are consistent with observations on the effect of blockers of specific mechanisms or receptors in patients with variant angina. Used alone, aspirin [10] (blocking thromboxane receptors), ketanserin [11] (blocking serotoninergic receptors) and phenotolamine [12] (blocking adrenergic receptors) do not prevent ischaemia because in each case alternative pathways remain active. However, if nitrates or calcium antagonists, which act directly on vascular smooth muscle, are employed, the response to all these stimuli is abolished, non-specifically.

Bertrand *et al.* [13] have examined the frequency of coronary artery spasm in response to methylergonovine in 1089 patients undergoing angiography. These authors showed that induced spasm is extremely common in patients with angina at rest and recent infarction but is very rare in stable angina, old infarction or atypical chest pain, which suggests that there may be an element of local vascular hyperreactivity in these acute coronary syndromes. It is possible that, in such circumstances, stimuli released from thrombi or some other source may provoke total occlusion in vessels, whereas in patients not liable to spasm occlusion is only partial. In addition, it may be speculated that other stimuli may exist that are so powerful as to provoke spasm in arteries irrespective of the vessels' inherent reactivity. Several recent studies have addressed this possibility.

Experimental studies

Clarke *et al.* [14] have studied neuropeptide Y and have shown that this peptide, in low concentrations in human coronary arteries, can induce myocardial ischaemia. This is the result not of constriction in the epicardial coronary arteries but of an effect on the resistance vessels that are too small to be angiographically visible. Of course this is a pharmacological study but it does show that constriction leading to ischaemia may take place in vessels that cannot be observed and as such, it carries the implication that lack of angiographically demonstrable constriction does not mean that constriction is not taking place.

Similar results have emerged from studies with endothelin in dogs by S.W. Larkin [15]. Doses as small as 3 pmol, injected into the left anterior descending artery of dogs, cause a reduction in blood flow and as the dose is increased to 100 pmol, flow drops pratically to zero. These reductions are accompanied by ischaemic changes in the ECG and, ultimately, ventricular fibrillation. Here too, however, no constriction was apparent in the epicardial coronary arteries; all the reduction in flow was attributable to more distal, resistance vessels not visible at angiography. *In vitro* studies by John Tippins [16], in arteries obtained from dogs and pigs, indicates that, compared to larger vessels, dose-response curves to vasoconstrictors are displaced to the left for smaller vessels. So it appears that different segments of coronary arteries respond differently to these agents.

Other interesting results are available from pharmacological studies. C.M. Newman showed that high dose acetylcholine causes considerable constriction in secondary and tertiary coronary arteries [17]. At low dose, however, it produces massive increases in coronary blood flow -increases of several hundred percent — through an action on resistance vessels. This contrasts with the results obtained by David Crossman which show that substance P which, at very tiny doses, causes massive dilatation of epicardial arteries but only a mild increase in blood flow [18].

Exactly what relevance such pharmacological studies hold for the pathology or pathophysiology of acute coronary syndrome must remain a matter of conjecture at present. However, it is apparent that coronary arteries have considerable potential for constriction and dilatation, depending on the circumstances. It is possible to speculate that an effect of constriction of either small or large vessels would be the promotion of stasis or the promotion of formation of a white thrombus which may progress to the occlusive red thrombus and which is the hallmark of coronary occlusion.

References

[1] Hackett D, Davies G, Chierchia S, Maseri A.
Intermittent coronary occlusion in acute myocardial infarction. Value of combined thrombolytic and vasodilator therapy.
N Engl J Med 1987; **63**: 1890–5.

[2] Hackett D, Davies G, Maseri A.
Coronary constriction in acute myocardial infarction: role of nitrates.
Eur Heart J 1988; **9** (suppl.A): 151–3.

[3] Vejar M, Hackett D, Brunelli C, *et al.* Comparison of low dose aspirin and coronary vasodilators in acute unstable angina. *Circulation* (in press).

[4] Vejar M, Fragasso G, Hackett D, *et al.* Dissociation of platelet activation and spontaneous myocardial ischaemia in unstable angina. *Thromb Haemos* 1990; **63:** 163–8.

[5] Hackett D, Larkin S, Chierchia S, Davies G, Kaski JC, Maseri A. Induction of coronary artery spasm by a direct local action of ergonovine. *Circulation* 1987; **75:** 577–82.

[6] Kaski JC, Maseri A, Vejar M, Crea F, Hackett D. Spontaneous coronary artery spasm in variant angina results from a local hyperreactivity to a generalized constrictor stimulus. *J Am Coll Cardiol* 1989; **14:** 1456–63.

[7] Maseri A, Davies G, Hackett D, Kaski JC. Coronary artery spasm and coronary vasoconstriction: the case for a distinction. *Circulation* (in press June 1990).

[8] Freedman B, Richmond DR, Kelly DT. Pathophysiology of coronary artery spasm. *Circulation* 1982; **66:** 705–9.

[9] Maseri A, Davies G, Hackett D, Kaski JC. Coronary artery spasm and coronary vasoconstriction: the case for a distinction. *Circulation* (in press).

[10] Chierchia S, Patrono C, Crea F, *et al.* Effects of intravenous prostacyclin in variant angina. *Circulation* 1982; **66:** 702–5.

[11] Freedman SB, Chierchia S, Rodriguez Plaza L, Bugiardini R, Smith G, Maseri A. Ergonovine-induced myocardial ischemia: no role for serotonergic receptors? *Circulation* 1984; **70:** 178–83.

[12] Chierchia S, Davies G, Berkenboom G, Crea F, Crean P, Maseri A. Alpha adrenergic receptors and coronary spasm: an elusive link. *Circulation* 1984; **69:** 8–14.

[13] Bertrand ME, La Blanche JM, Tilmant PY, *et al.* Frequency of provoked coronary arterial spasm in 1089 consecutive patients undergoing coronary arteriography. *Circulation* 1982; **65:** 1299–306.

[14] Clarke JG, Davies GJ, Kerwin R, *et al.* Coronary artery infusion of neuropeptide Y in patients with angina pectoris. *Lancet* 1987; **i:** 1057–9.

[15] Larkin SW, Clarke JG, Keogh BE, *et al.* Intracoronary endothelin induces myocardial ischemia by small vessel constriction in the dog. *Am J Cardiol* 1989; **64:** 956–8.

[16] Tippins JR, Antoniw JW, Maseri A. Endothelin-1 is a potent constrictor in conductive and resistive coronary arteries. *J Cardiovasc Pharma* 1989; **13**(suppl.5): S211–2.

[17] Newman CM, Hackett DR, Fryer M, El-Tamimi HM, Davies GJ, Maseri A. Dual effects of acetylcholine on angiographically normal human coronary arteries *in vivo*. [Abstract] *Circulation* 1987; **76**(suppl.IV): 56.

[18] Crossman DC, Larkin SW, Fuller RW, Davies GJ, Maseri A. Substance P dilates epicardial coronary arteries and increases coronary blood flow in humans. *Circulation* 1989; **80:** 475–84.

2. DIAGNOSTIC METHODS IN ACUTE ISCHAEMIA

ANTIMYOSIN ANTIBODIES

W.S. HILLIS

Antimyosin antibodies as non-invasive markers of myocardial necrosis

Several radiopharmaceuticals are available which are sequestered by acutely infarcting myocardium. The regions of increased myocardial uptake are useful in the detection, localization and quantification of necrosis. These agents are particularly valuable when other indirect techniques for measuring the extent of irreversible tissue damage have associated technical limitations secondary to specific clinical presentations. Potential uses might include: after late admission with chest pain when typical electrocardiographic changes may have reversed to a degree, and when an elevation of cardiac enzymes may be missed; following bypass grafting, where enzyme release may be very similar to that found in myocardial infarction; where localization of necrosis is difficult due to ECG abnormalities such as conduction defects or the presence of Wolff-Parkinson-White syndrome; and, finally, as a marker of infarct size after thrombolytic therapy, where typical creatine phosphokinase (CPK) release curves may be altered quantitatively and qualitatively in the presence of coronary artery reperfusion.

Experimental studies

The first use of radiolabelled antimyosin antibodies was reported by Khaw *et al.* in 1976 [1], in a canine experimental model of myocardial infarction. Following the administration of non-specific antimyosin antibodies, the dogs were sacrificed and antibody uptake was measured at the infarct centre, sub-dividing this into endo and epicardial regions, the former being the more vulnerable zone to myocardial ischaemic changes. The uptake of antibodies in these regions was compared to corresponding normal tissues. An uptake ratio of 4:1 was found at the infarct centre. When intravenous doses of I-125 labelled antimyosin $(Fab')_2$ fragments were administered after 72 hours of coronary occlusion, it was shown that the relative specificity of antibody uptake for endocardium in the infarct centre compared to equivalent normal tissue was 14:1.

Khaw *et al.* [2] extended their work by the use of radioactive labelled microspheres in dogs. These spheres are similar in size to red blood cells and are distributed in the myocardium in the ratio of blood flow. It was demonstrated that uptake of antimyosin antibodies was inversely related to blood flow (Fig. 1), suggesting that uptake of antibody was a relatively good marker reflecting reduction in coronary flow to the critical degree leading to myocardial necrosis. There was also a good histological correlation with the degree of antibody uptake.

Further studies by this group [3] showed that in the early phase of developing infarction (up to 24 hours) there was a much greater uptake of technetium pyrophosphate than of antimyosin antibodies by infarcted tissue. When uptake was related to blood flow, however, it became apparent that the uptake of antimyosin antibody showed a linear, inverse relationship to regional blood flow, whereas technetium pyrophosphate was taken up by myocardium with reductions of regional

Fig. 1. This graph shows the relationship between ^{131}I-Ab(Fab')₂ localization in infarcted myocardium and corresponding regional blood flow measured using radioactive microspheres 72 hours after coronary occlusion in a canine model. (Reproduced with permission from Khaw BA, Beller GA, Haber E. *Circulation* 1977; **57**: 750. [2])

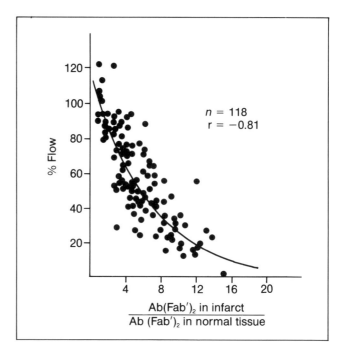

blood flow of 31%-50%, suggesting that pyrophosphate may overestimate absolute infarct size.

Subsequent studies in dogs subjected to occlusion and reperfusion showed there were very high uptake ratios for antimyosin antibodies in the myocardium of dogs in which reperfusion occurred, suggesting that antibody uptake may be a particularly sensitive index in animal models studying reperfusion as well as ischaemia. Frame *et al* [4] also studied antibody uptake in dogs subject to occlusion and reperfusion and their results indicated that uptake might be a useful measurement of serial change in the myocardium in the aftermath of reperfusion, and may offer a means of assessing reperfusion damage and its modulation by pharmacological interventions.

Clinical studies

Braat *et al.* [5] examined 31 patients with chest pain of >30 minutes duration, new Q-waves and elevated enzymes and found that 17 out of 17 anterior infarctions could be localized by three planar images following radiolabelled antibody injection at 24 hours. Visualization at 48 hours was not superior to the earlier image. The same group used technetium labelled antibodies in conjunction with single photon emission computed tomography (SPECT), to evaluate the length of the hypokinetic segment and compared the results with those obtained by ventriculograms taken 10-14 days post-myocardial infarction [6]. There was good correlation (r=0.79, P<0.002) between the two techniques (Fig. 2). The size of the infarct measured by technetium pyrophosphate was 1.7 times greater than that observed with antimyosin antibodies. One suggested explanation for this is that the uptake of antibodies specifically reflects necrotic damage, whereas technetium may also be taken up by a superficial layer of tissue with potentially reversible ischaemic damage. If correct, serial measurements with both scanning agents may be valuable in assessing infarct reduction following coronary artery reperfusion.

Antunes *et al.* [7] used indium 111 labelled antimyosin antibodies to examine 35 patients. Adequate images were not obtained in eight patients, and it is possible that

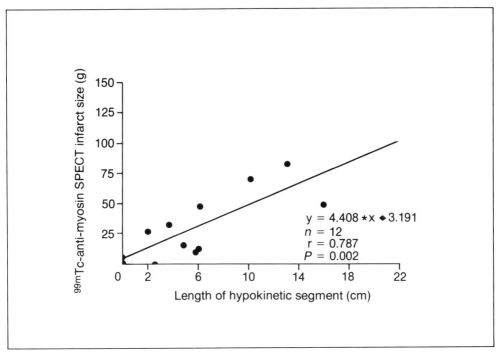

Fig. 2. This graph shows the infarct weight in grams estimated by antimyosin SPECT on the vertical axis, with the hypokinetic segment length on the horizontal axis. (Reproduced with permission from Khaw BA, Gold HK, Yasuda T, *et al. Circulation* 1986; **74:** 501–8. [6])

this particular technique may not be as widely applicable as was previously suggested on the basis of earlier pilot studies. There was, however, good correlation between infarct size as assessed by the antibody/SPECT method, and ejection fraction 10-14 days post-myocardial infarction (r=0.71, P<0.01). There was also a good correlation with individual regional wall motion scores. In this study, 19 patients had received thrombolytic therapy and reperfusion occurred in 11. In those in whom reperfusion was not achieved, a reasonable correlation (r=0.66) was demonstrated between infarct size, as estimated by antibody uptake, and peak CK values. There was also a good correlation between infarct size as indicated by indium-labelled antibody and infarct size, determined by technetium pyrophosphate.

Volpini *et al.* [8] looked at infarct size determined by indium labelled antimyosin antibodies and compared these to the traditional non-invasive techniques for the measurement of infarct size, comparing electrocardiographic indices, infarct size as assessed by technetium pyrophosphate and left ventriculography. They showed an excellent correlation with all these standard indices in terms of diagnosis and localization of infarction (Fig. 3).

The advantages of the antibody technique include its rapid blood pool clearance, high target-to-background ratio, and the fact that the antibody is not taken up by overlying tissue, as may occur with other 'hot-spotting' agents. Against this, hepatic uptake may mask small inferior infarcts.

Finally, several groups have measured the release of myosin light chains in serum following myocardial damage using antimyosin antibodies *in vitro*. This may be helpful as a diagnostic test when other non-invasive indices are inappropriate. Katus *et al.* [9] have undertaken studies which suggest that the presence of myosin

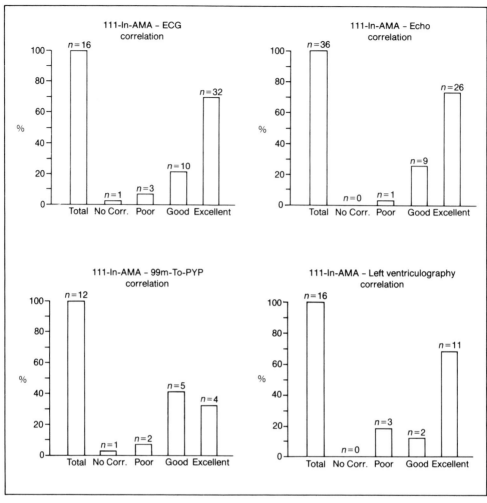

Fig. 3. These block diagrams confirm the accuracy of AMA-Fab in defining extent and localization of infarction compared with electrocardiographic, echocardiographic, technetium-99m pyrophosphate scintigraphic and left ventriculographic studies. (Reproduced with permission from Volpini M, Giubbini R, Gei P, *et al. Am J Cardiol* 1989; **63**: 7–13. [8])

light chains in serum is highly specific for the diagnosis of myocardial infarction. The time scale of light chain release differs from that of CPK (Fig. 4), light chain release starting later after infarction with a much later peak. The application of this technique may be appropriate in assessing late myocardial damage and remodelling following infarction.

Conclusion

The potential displayed from the use of antimyosin antibodies in animal studies appears to have been substantiated in human studies. Myocardial antibody uptake is related to tissue necrosis, and clinical studies confirm infarct localization. Comparative studies with other radionuclides may suggest other applications for antimyosin antibodies, not least in the evaluation of the effectiveness of coronary thrombolysis and reperfusion.

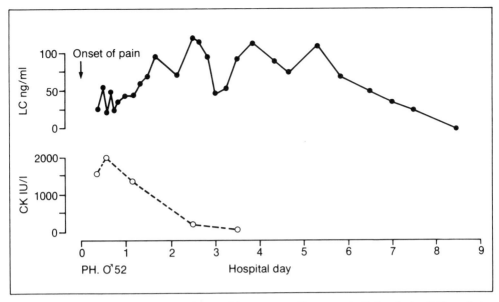

Fig. 4. These graphs show the release of human cardiac myosin light chain (LC) and the corresponding serum creatine kinase (CK) activity from a patient with acute myocardial infarction obtained over a period of 8.5 days. (Reproduced with permission from Katus HA, Yasuda T, Gold HK, *et al. Am J Cardiol* 1984; **54**: 964–70. [9])

References

[1] Khaw BA, Beller GA, Haber E, Smith TW.
Localization of cardiac myosin-specific
antibody in myocardial infarction.
J Clin Invest 1976: **58**: 439–46.

[2] Khaw BA, Beller GA, Haber E.
Experimental myocardial infarct imaging
following intravenous administration of
Iodine-131 labeled antibody (Fab-)2
fragments specific for cardiac myosin.
Circulation 1977: **57**: 750.

[3] Beller GA, Khaw BA, Haber E, Smith TW.
Localization of radiolabeled cardiac myosin-
specific antibody in myocardial infarcts.
Comparison with Technetium-99m stannous
pyrophosphate.
Circulation 1977: **55**: 74–8.

[4] Frame LH, Lopez A, Khaw BA, Fallon J,
Haber E, Powell WJ.
Early membrane damage during coronary
reperfusion in dogs. Detection by
radiolabeled anticardiac myosin (Fab-)2.
J Clin Invest 1983: **72**: 535–44.

[5] Braat SH, de Zwaan C, Teule J, Heidenal G,
Wellens HJJ.
Value of Indium-111 monoclonal
antimyosin antibody for imaging in acute
myocardial infarction.
Am J Cardiol 1987: **60**: 725–6.

[6] Khaw BA, Gold HK, Yasuda T, *et al.*
Scintigraphic quantification of myocardial
necrosis in patients after intravenous
injection of myosin-specific antibody.
Circulation 1986; **74**: 501–8.

[7] Antunes ML, Seldin DW, Wall RM,
Johnson LL.
Measurement of acute Q-wave myocardia!
infarct size with single photon emission
computed tomography imaging of Indium-
111 antimyosin.
Am J Cardiol 1989; **63**: 777–83.

[8] Volpini M, Giubbini R, Gei P, *et al.*
Diagnosis of acute myocardial infarction by
Indium-111 antimyosin antibodies and
correlation with the traditional techniques
for the evaluation of extent and localization.
Am J Cardiol 1989; **63**: 7–13.

[9] Katus HA, Yasuda T, Gold HK, *et al.*
Diagnosis of acute myocardial infarction by
detection of circulating cardiac myosin light
chains.
Am J Cardiol 1984; **54**: 964–70.

MAGNETIC RESONANCE IMAGING

A.L. MUIR

The relaxation parameters that can be measured by magnetic resonance imaging (MRI) have been shown to be abnormal in the variety of conditions where there is an excess of water. It has therefore been speculated that it may be possible to document the changes that follow myocardial infarction, and perhaps myocardial ischaemia, with MRI.

MRI in myocardial infarction

In 1985, we demonstrated that the relaxation parameter T_1 was increased after myocardial infarction and this allowed imaging of the infarcted tissue (Been *et al.*). Fig. 1 is a coronal section from a man who sustained an inferior myocardial infarction eight days prior to imaging. The picture clearly shows a pericardial effusion, which is very common after myocardial infarction, but in addition both ventricles may be discerned and on the inferior wall of the left ventricle an area of increased density representing the area of infarction.

A review of the literature on human and animal studies reveals that investigators have looked at two different parameters of magnetic resonance relaxation, T_1 and T_2. Two different types of pulse sequence are used in these studies — spin-echo and inversion recovery — and the choice of sequence has a significant bearing on the results obtained. T_1 is measured more readily by inversion recovery, T_2 more easily by the spin-echo method. Indeed, in several studies, the choice of technique has effectively limited researchers to measuring either T_1 or T_2. This reflects the different natures of T_1 and T_2. When nuclei are subjected to a magnetic field, they adopt a regular orientation. This can be disrupted by the passage of a pulse of radio waves. Their subsequent

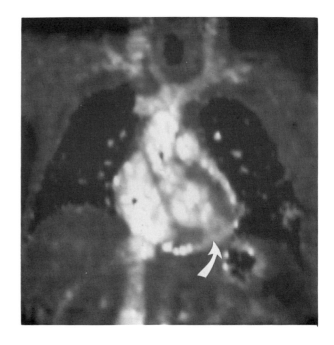

Fig. 1. Gated T_1 coronal image of a man eight days after inferior myocardial infarction. The infarcted heart shows an area of high T_1 in the intero-apical region of the left ventricle above the arrow. There is also a small amount of pericardial fluid seen as a rim of very high T_1. (Reproduced with permission from Been M, Smith MA, Ridgeway JP, *et al. Lancet* 1985; **ii:** 348–50. [1])

return to equilibrium is an exponential process described by the time constant T_1, often referred to as 'spin-lattice' relaxation time. T_2 is somewhat different. Each nucleus exerts a magnetic influence over neighbouring nuclei; radiowave perturbation prompts 'spin-spin' interactions and leads to 'dephasing' of nuclei as some speed up and others slow down. The subsequent return to equilibrium is again an exponential process, described by the time constant T_2.

Fig. 2 shows the sort of image that may be obtained with the inversion recovery technique. It comes from a man who had suffered a septal infarction and it provides a colour-keyed indication of T_1 values. In the affected area of the ventricle, T_1 is about 400 msec; in normal ventricle, T_1 is in the range 300-320 msec. We have recorded similar values in nearly 100 patients; other workers will probably get slightly different values, depending on their measurement techniques. But our data concerning measurements of T_1 conform very well to existing MRC standards for this technique.

Fig. 3 shows normal and abnormal values of T_1 in a patient with an inferior infarct. In general, it has proved easier to study inferior infarcts with coronal rather than transverse projection.

MRI permits three-dimensional imaging of an infarct and it has been possible to compare the volume of the infarct estimated in this way with peak plasma levels of creatine kinase (CK). There is quite a reasonable correlation, and this also holds good for the total area under the time/concentration curve for CK. We have also compared infarct volumes as estimated by MRI with values obtained using the technetium pyrophosphate/SPECT technique and have found a good correlation between the

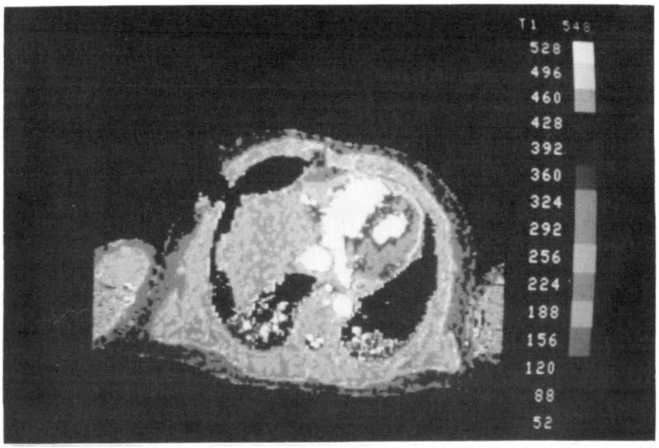

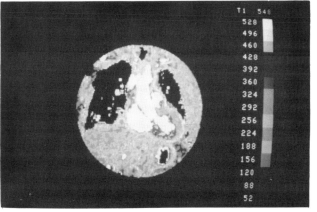

Fig. 2. Transverse section of thorax from a patient who has sustained a recent septal infarct. Septal areas show T_1 values >400 msec.

Fig. 3. Coronal section of thorax from a patient who has sustained a recent inferior infarct. Note the T_1 values >400 msec along inferior margin.

two techniques (r = 6.9) in this group of patients (Fig. 4). Given the technical difficulties attending both procedures, this is quite a good result.

What is the time course of the changes seen on MRI after infarction? Theory, and the results of experimental work, suggest that abnormalities should be apparent early [1-4]. We examined this proposition in 20 normal controls and 41 patients with first infarcts [5]. All were free of failure at the time of imaging and in stable cardiac rhythm — essential for the use of electrocardiographic gating. Whenever possible images were taken on day 1-3, 4-7 and 8-14 post-infarction, and then monthly for six months.

The results were unexpected (Fig. 5). Representative trends in T_1 are shown in Fig. 6. It is apparent that, while there is an increase in T_1 on the third day post-infarction, peak abnormal T_1 is reached only at about day 14. The values are still grossly abnormal one month after infarction. Normal T_1 values are not restored until some five or six months after infarction. If oedema alone was a signal, a much earlier, steeper increase in T_1 values might have been expected; Fig. 6 relates the pattern of T_1 changes to known changes in the heart following infarction. Plainly, oedema alone cannot account for the T_1 variations observed. This finding adds to disappointments with MRI in some other areas. Even in animal studies, changes in the myocardium cannot be discerned earlier than two hours after infarction. The overall conclusion to be drawn from this appears to be that, at least with present MRI technology, the procedure cannot be used to evaluate very early changes in the infarcted heart.

Future developments

In animal studies, results have been improved by the use of paramagnetic contrast enhancing agents. We have had no experience with such agents in cardiological practice, but have used them in neurology wherein the administration of gadolinium improves the resolution. Results from animal studies indicate that this approach may well enhance the imaging of myocardial infarction. However, it appears to discriminate poorly between ischaemic and infarcted tissue and the results from animal studies are still somewhat conflicting. Other contrast agents are being investigated.

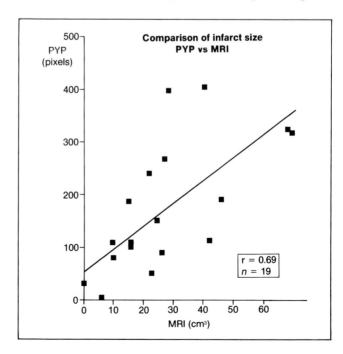

Fig. 4. A comparison of infarct volume assessed by magnetic resonance imaging and by 99mTc pyrophosphate SPECT imaging.

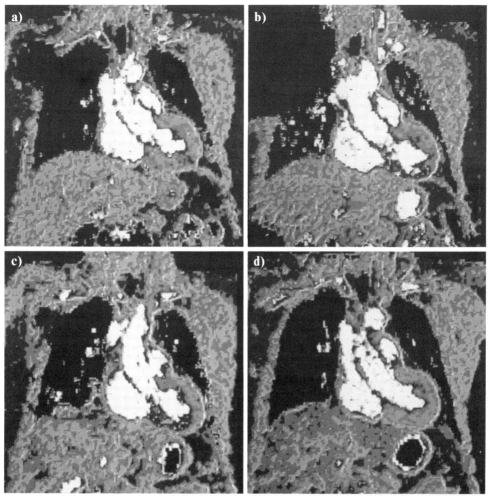

Fig. 5. Sequential coronal images in a patient with inferior infarction: (a) three days, (b) 14 days, (c) one month, and (d) three months after infarction. (Reproduced with permission from Been M, Smith MA, Ridgeway JP, *et al. Br Heart J* 1988; **59**: 1–8. [5])

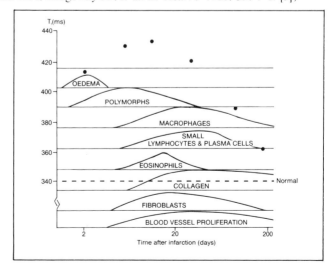

Fig. 6. Plot of T_1 changes with time after infarction contrasted with known histological changes.

41

The use of such contrast agents may turn out to be the way of the future, but another avenue that deserves consideration is spectroscopy. Bottomley [6] has studied four patients with acute infarction using this technique, and has recorded changes in phosphocreatinine and inorganic phosphate consistent with acute infarction. At present there are problems with the localization of the spectroscopic signal, but if these can be overcome this may offer a new and very exciting way of looking more closely at the events of acute myocardial infarction.

References

[1] Been M, Smith MA, Ridgeway JP, et al.
Characterisation of acute myocardial
infarction by gated magnetic resonance
imaging.
Lancet 1985; ii: 348–50.

[2] Mather-De Vre R.
Biomedical implications of the relaxation
behaviour of water related to NMR imaging.
Br J Radiol 1984; 57: 955–76.

[3] Williams ES, Kaplan JL, Thatcher F,
Zimmerman G, Knoebel SB.
Prolongation of proton spin-lattice
relaxation times in regionally ischaemic
tissue from dog hearts.
J Nucl Med 1980; 21: 449–53.

[4] Higgins CB, Herfkens R, Lipton MJ, et al.
Nuclear magnetic resonance imaging of
acute myocardial infarction in dogs:
alterations in magnetic relaxation times.
Am J Cardiol 1983; 52: 184–8.

[5] Been M, Smith MA, Ridgeway JP, et al.
Serial changes in the T_1 magnetic relaxation
parameter after myocardial infarction in
man.
Br Heart J 1988; 59: 1–8.

[6] Bottomley PA, Herekens RJ, Smith LS,
Bashore TM.
Altered phosphate metabolism in
myocardial infarction: P31 MR
spectroscopy.
Radiology 1987; 165: 703–7.

WHOLE HEART PET STUDIES FOR CLINICAL RESEARCH

L. ARAUJO, T. JONES, A. MASERI

Introduction

Positron emission tomography (PET) is a nuclear medicine technique that allows quantification of radioactivity within the body *in vivo*. This differentiates it from single photon tomography, even with three-dimensional reconstruction, which cannot provide true quantification.

This technique involves the use of positrons which are isotopes with a very short half-life which therefore have to be produced in site by a particle accelerator machine called a cyclotron. The procedure is very complex, relying on the external detection of positron release in the body. The technique is also in a state of considerable flux with new advances and improvements occurring rapidly. This is exemplified by the PET scanner currently in use at the MRC Cyclotron Unit at the Hammersmith Hospital. This machine, used for three-dimensional imaging, has a spatial resolution of 6 mm. One of its relatively recent predecessors had a resolution of 16 mm; spatial resolution of three-dimensional single photon emission computed tomography (SPECT) offers a resolution of about 20 mm. Prices that have to be paid for such high quality images are the considerable cost of the equipment and set-up, and a certain amount of patient discomfort as a study may take a long time to generate the images, during which period the patient has to remain still.

The process by which images are generated is technically complex as it involves sophisticated computers and software. It is important to remember, however, that because the process is quantitative it is possible to correct for background activity and so obtain high resolution images which provide true quantifiable information in the regions of interest. This process is exemplified in Figs. 1 and 2. In Fig. 1, the first image

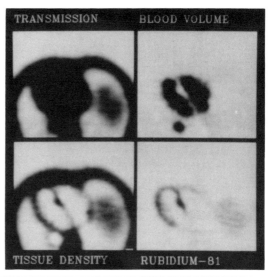

Fig. 1. PET studies can be used to generate high resolution images providing quantifiable information on regions of interest by subtracting one image from another.

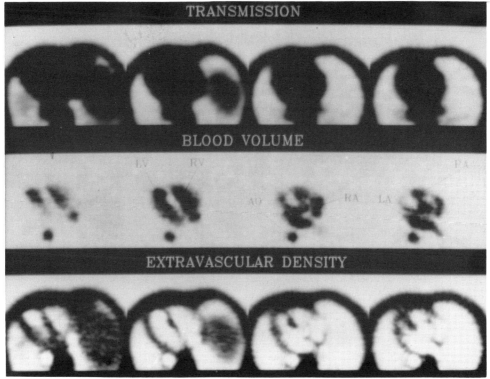

Fig. 2. Multiple cross-sectional images of the heart can be obtained for use in 3-D reconstruction.

is a transmission image showing the lungs, liver and heart. The blood volume image was obtained using the blood-pool tracer $C^{15}O$ (half-life two minutes). The aorta, septum and all four chambers of the heart may be discerned. Superimposing these images and subtracting one from the other results in a tissue density image which is shown in the bottom left panel. The atrial and ventricular septa, attachment of the papillary muscles, walls of both ventricles, aorta and spine may be seen. Tissue density may be calculated in a similar way for each element in the image, be it blood flow, tissue metabolism or receptor binding sites, so providing a quantitative analysis of these features. The last image of Fig. 1 shows the rubidium concentration in the heart walls and represents the mass of heart muscle present in each region. Fig. 2 shows similar images to Fig. 1 and illustrates the possibility of obtaining multiple cross-sectional images of the heart which can be used for 3-D reconstruction.

An instance of the application of this approach is illustrated in Fig. 3. It shows regional coronary blood flow as calculated by PET compared to estimates obtained from microsphere studies which were used as a 'gold standard' independent method. There is remarkably good agreement between the two techniques.

PET studies of cardiac pathology

Workers at the Hammersmith Hospital have undertaken a range of studies, using PET to examine aspects of cardiac physiology and pathology that may be evaluated by other means, in order to get an idea of how useful PET is for making these measurements. In patients with chronic stable angina,PET has been used to measure blood flow in areas of normal myocardium and areas distal to stenosis. It has also been possible to compare blood flow in normal myocardium and in situations of successful and unsuccessful thrombolysis post-myocardial infarction. As would be predicted, blood flow was lower when thrombolysis failed than when thrombolysis succeeded.

Using three-dimensional PET images, it is possible to distinguish between ischaemic and necrotic myocardial tissue. Using water labelled with ^{15}O, it is possible to identify areas of myocardium in which blood flow after myocardial infarction may be perhaps 40% below normal. Subsequently, rubidium tracer is administered in

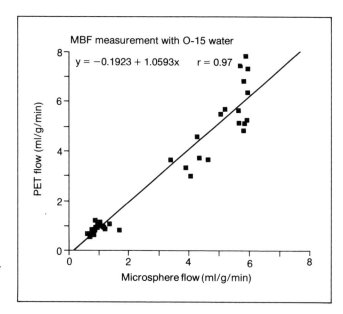

Fig. 3. Correlation between regional coronary blood flow calculated by PET and by microspheres studies.

order to characterise the myocardial tissue with low blood flow. This is taken up by cells in amounts proportionate to intracellular potassium content. While necrotic tissue loses much of its potassium, a greater amount is retained in ischaemic tissues. Hence, when the images of blood flow and potassium content are superimposed, it is possible to identify areas of myocardium which, despite their greatly reduced blood flow, are still viable and may be salvaged.

Another application of the technique is the evaluation of ischaemia following dipyridamole administration in patients with coronary artery stenosis. In normal tissues supplied by normal arteries, administration of dipyridamole may enhance blood flow three-fold or more. Overall blood flow to tissues supplied by stenotic vessels is increased only very slightly and, because of drug-induced transmural steal, there is actually a reduction in supply to endocardial tissues, with resulting ischaemia. The tracer 18-deoxyglucose is preferentially taken up by ischaemic tissue, so if this is administered after dipyridamole challenge it is possible to demonstrate the extent and exact distribution of the myocardium in jeopardy as a result of coronary artery disease.

PET is a relatively new technique and the experience gained with it is necessarily limited. It has tremendous potential, however, and development proceeds apace. It is already apparent that it can be used to replicate findings from existing modes of investigation and also to provide information unobtainable by other means. One area of growing interest is its application to the study of myocardial beta receptors. It is sure to become increasingly important as a non-invasive means of evaluating cardiac physiology and pathology.

CAN INFARCT SIZE AND ITS MODIFICATION BE MEASURED IN MAN? THE CASE FOR

K. SWEDBERG

Introduction

A method that measures infarct size in the clinical situation should ideally be non-invasive, preferrably cheap and simple, and should be suitable for use in coronary care units. Furthermore, to be of real practical use it should also give rapid results. No existing method fulfils all these requirements, and accordingly several complementary methods are necessary. In addition, it is reasonable to assume that larger infarcts are associated with higher mortality and morbidity than smaller ones, and the methods should reflect this. From the clinician's point of view, it is essential that this kind of assumption be taken into consideration.

In principle, electrocardiography (ECG), enzyme release profiles, vectorcardiography, echocardiography, radioisotope angiography, computerized tomography, magnetic resonance imaging and positron emission tomography may all be used to evaluate infarct size, but if the 'clinician's criterion' is applied this list may be shortened to ECG findings, enzyme release profiles and radioisotope angiography. The remainder of this presentation will therefore concentrate on these three techniques.

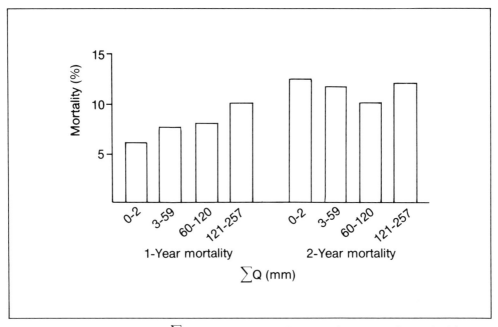

Fig. 1. Relationship between $\sum Q$ in the 24 precordial leads four days after arrival in hospital in anterior myocardial infarction, and 1- and 2-year mortality ($P > 0.2$) rates. Patients divided into quartiles according to final $\sum Q$. ($n = 197$; n in each quartile from left: 48, 51, 49, 49.) (Reproduced with permission from Herlitz J, Hjalmarsson Å. *Clin Cardiol* 1985; **8**: 141–7. [1])

Electrocardiographic studies
When using the ECG, it is assumed that the development of Q-waves provides some indication of infarct-size and that elevation of the ST segment reflects ischaemic muscle mass. If correct this would be an ideal situation. However, studies using a 24-electrode mapping technique, that provides much more information than standard ECG, cast doubt on this assumption. Fig. 1 shows data, first presented by John Herlitz in 1984 from our first Gothenburg metoprolol trial [1], in which the development of Q-waves over the first four post-infarction days in victims of first infarction was related to later morbidity and mortality. Clearly, there is no relation between ECG changes and long term outcome. Further work in this field has emphasized that ECG changes do not adequately reflect infarct size.

Electrical changes in the heart may be of some value in this respect, and we are at present evaluating the usefulness of computerized vectorcardiography at the Department of Medicine, University of Gothenburg. It will, however, be some time before firm pronouncements can be made about the value of this technique.

Plasma protein markers
Enzyme release profiles seem more promising for the determination of infarct size. Creatine kinase (CK) and lactate dehydrogenase (LDH) are released by necrotic myocardium and can be detected in the blood by simple analyses. For diagnostic purposes, the specificity of this technique might be enhanced by assaying specific isoenzymes of LDH or CK. When Sobel, in 1972, proposed measurement of CK as a means of calculating infarct size, he was able to show a relationship between infarct size and morbidity/mortality, larger infarcts being associated with a higher incidence of mor-

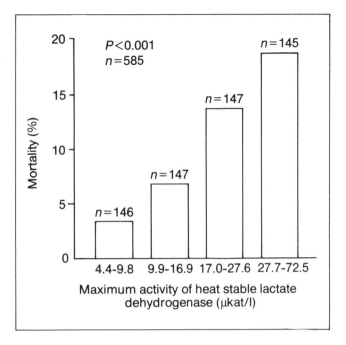

Fig. 2. Correlation between maximum activity of heat stable lactate dehydrogenase and three month mortality in all patients. (Reproduced with permission from Herlitz J, Hjalmarsson Å, Waldenström J, Swedberg K, Waagstein F, Waldenström A. *Br Heart J* 1983; **50:** 520–4.]4])

tality [2]. Thompson *et al.* from Australia reported similar findings — mortality was related to infarct size, and mortality over one year was also related to peak plasma CK [3].

In our own study, conducted among 580 patients with first myocardial infarction, mortality at three months and one year was significantly associated with release of heat-stable LDH (Fig. 2) [4]. Release of LDH was also related to duration of pain — a widely used clinical guide to ischaemia — and also to the three-month incidence of heart failure. Enzymes, then, appear to be clincially useful indicators of infarct size.

Radioisotope angiography

This also appears potentially useful. In a study in 19 patients, Wackers *et al.* were able to demonstrate a relation between infarct size as estimated by angiography and infarct size at autopsy (Fig. 3) [5]. Johnson *et al.*, in a dog model, evaluated infarct size using antimyosin antibodies (Fab fragments) labelled with indium-111 with single photon emission computed tomography (SPECT) [6]. They, too, found very good agreement between estimated infarct size and actual size as determined post-mortem. When used in conjunction with thallium-201 images, the data obtained from this antibody study could be used to estimate the percentage of infarcted myocardium; here again, agreement with post-mortem data was excellent. Several other studies, using different isotopes, have confirmed these findings. Botvinick *et al.* have also shown good correlation between estimated infarct size, morbidity and mortality [7].

Dr Ann Tweddel and colleagues at Glasgow have shown that infarct size may be estimated using a gated tomography technique with thallium-201 [8,9]. They have developed an index that relates infarct perfusion defect to infarct size (as determined at autopsy in 22 patients). By integrating this with the Norris index, they were able to relate estimated infarct size to prognosis, the former providing an indication of the latter.

Fig. 3. Relationship between size of infarction determined on the basis of postmortem findings and size of scintigraphically abnormal area as calculated by computer processing of schematic drawing of thallium-201 scintiscans (CSC%). The dotted lines indicate shift of the regression line by 10% of the total left ventricle. N = 19; r = 0.91 for anterior infarcts; r = 0.97 for inferior infarcts; r = 0.86 for anterior-inferior infarcts. Abbreviations: CHF = congestive heart failure; LV = left ventricle. (Reproduced with permission from Wackers F, Becker A, Samson G, *et al. Circulation* 1977; **56:** 72–8. [5])

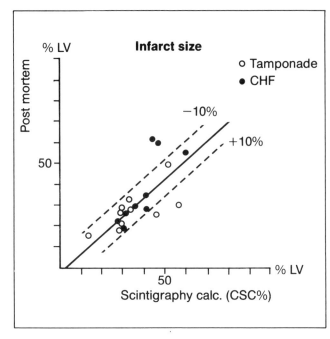

Conclusion

I believe it is possible to measure infarct size in a clinical setting. Of still greater value, however, would be the ability to estimate the amount of ischaemic myocardium in the early stages of developing acute myocardial infarction. Progress in this sphere must await the emergence of new methods of investigation.

References

[1] Herlitz J, Hjalmarsson Å. The relationship between the electrocardiographically estimated infarct size and 1- and 2 year survival in acute myocardial infarction. *Clin Cardiol* 1985; **8:** 141–7.

[2] Sobel E, Bresnahan G, Shell W, Yoder R. Estimation of infarct size in man and its relation to prognosis. *Circulation* 1972; **XLVI:** 640–8.

[3] Thompson P, Fletcher E, Katavatis V. Enzymatic indices of myocardial necrosis: influence on short- and long-term prognosis after myocardial infarction. *Circulation* 1979; **59:** 113–9.

[4] Herlitz J, Hyalmarsson Å, Waldenström J, Swedberg K, Waagstein F, Waldenström A. Correlation between enzymatically estimated infarct size and early mortality rate. *Br Heart J* 1983; **50:** 520–4.

[5] Wackers F, Becker A, Samson G, *et al.* Location and size of acute transmural myocardial infarction estimated from thallium-201 scintiscans. *Circulation* 1977; **56:** 72–8.

[6] Johnson L, Lerrick K, Coromilas J, *et al.* Measurement of infarct size and percentage myocardium infarcted in a dog preparation with single photon-emission computed tomography, thallium-201, and indium 111-monoclonal antimyosin Fab. *Circulation* 1987; **76:** 181–90.

[7] Botvinick E, Perez-Gonzalez J, Dunn R, *et al.* Late prognostic value of scintigraphic parameters of acute myocardial infarction size in complicated myocardial infarction without heart failure. *Am J Cardiol* 1983; **7:** 1045–51.

[8] Tweddel A, *et al.* Acute perfusion imaging for infarct size. *Eur Heart J* 1988; **9** (suppl.): 212.

[9] Tweddel A. Personal communication.

CAN INFARCT SIZE AND ITS MODIFICATION BE MEASURED IN MAN? THE CASE AGAINST

D.J. HEARSE

For 20 years, experimentalists have studied infarct size and claimed many interventions to be protective. It is paradoxical that nowadays, clinicians are claiming successful drug-induced limitation of infarct size [1] while experimentalists are doubting the concept and are even questioning our ability to adequately measure infarct size and its limitation [2].

In addressing the question of whether or not infarct size can be measured in the clinical setting, it could be argued that knowledge of ultimate infarct size *per se* is of little real use to the physician and that even if this information were available it would make little difference to the treatment of patients, or to their prognosis.

Factors determining infarct size

As a prelude to a discussion of whether or not infarct size can be measured in man, it is essential to consider the baseline variables that determine infarct size. These variables are fairly well defined:

1. The volume of the ischaemic zone (the 'risk zone');
2. The extent of residual or collateral flow to the risk zone;
3. The values of various haemodynamic parameters, such as rate-pressure product, that influence metabolic demand within the tissues of the ischaemic zone.

As has been shown so clearly in the AMPIM study [3], these critical baseline predictors *must* be taken into account when evaluating infarct size and its modification.

The volume of the ischaemic zone at risk of infarction is a simple anatomical factor. It depends on the site of the occlusion and on the anatomic size of the perfusion bed served by the occluded vessel. Both these factors are highly variable between individuals and, as a consequence, it is extremely difficult to make comparisons between hearts or simply to predict the likely size of an infarct. This variability makes it even more difficult to assess the ability of any intervention to alter infarct size. In any drug trial, where it is not possible to determine the site of occlusion or the anatomy of the vessels, simple comparisons of the infarct size are difficult and potentially misleading.

Residual blood flow may be delivered from a variety of sources. It may come from adjoining perfusion beds, via anastomoses between adjacent coronary vessels (the so-called 'coronary collaterals'); some nutrient flow to the ischaemic zone may arise from venous retroperfusion; and, finally, there may be some residual flow via a partial stenosis. All of these sources of residual blood flow are highly variable, particularly the collateral connections which differ greatly not only between hearts but also between different areas in the same heart. I would argue that it is not possible to compare infarct size between groups without taking account of the effects of residual flow.

Residual nutrient flow to tissue at risk of infarction may exert some very important effects upon that tissue. First, it may act to salvage tissue within the ischaemic risk zone, so that the extent of infarction is reduced and a non-transmural infarction will result. In other words, a natural form of infarct size limitation may well occur. The

49

extent of residual flow is also going to be an important determinant of the speed at which the tissue infarcts. Such highly variable factors make comparison of infarct size between different hearts very difficult, particularly if assessments are carried out at different times.

It is my proposition that in any study of the effects of an intervention on infarct size, it is not sufficient simply to measure ultimate infarct size. It is essential to measure, and correct for, the influences of the baseline determinants described above. If one has a knowledge of these indices then it is possible to use the 'salvage index' in order to predict accurately the ultimate size of an evolving infarct [2,4]. Thus, if we want to assess the effects of drugs or reperfusion on infarct size we should be addressing ourselves not merely to measuring infarct size, but also to measuring these vital baseline variables with sufficient precision to make meaningful interpretations.

Measuring infarct size

As far as the first of these aims is concerned, Dr Swedberg has touched on several methods that may be used to *estimate* the volume or mass of infarcted tissue (see page 45). I maintain that in the clinical arena creatine kinase estimation and/or electrocardiogram analysis are imprecise methods which are prone to artifacts. While they may distinguish between big infarcts and small infarcts, and may even indicate the directionality of damage or a change in size of an infarct, I do not believe that these techniques can measure a 10% or 20% change in infarct size (which is the scale of change that may be hoped for with some interventions). Current imaging techniques are still of insufficient power, resolution or definition to be able to measure precisely infarct size. It seems to me that, in man, infarct size really can still only be measured at post mortem; even then, it is far from easy, particularly in the presence of diffuse ischaemia.

Measuring baseline variables

What about measurement of the two most important determinants of infarct size, namely the size of area at risk and the extent of collateral or residual flow? While risk zone size can be estimated in experimental animals, the techniques used (injection of microspheres or dyes) cannot be routinely applied to the human heart. I would maintain that at the present time, the risk zone size cannot adequately be quantified in patients. Even techniques such as positron emission tomography, which may one day provide a solution to this problem, do not yet offer sufficient precision.

Measurement of collateral or residual flow, a crucial determinant of infarct size, again can be achieved in animals through the use of radioactive markers but in man means do not exist to provide a precise measurement of flow distribution within the ischaemic zone.

Conclusion

While we remain unable to measure such variables as size of ischaemic risk zone and the extent of collateral flow in man, we cannot make any reliable calculations regarding infarct size or changes in infarct size in response to various interventions.

References

[1] Herlitz J, Hjalmarson A.
The role of beta blockade in the limitation of infarct development.
Eur Heart J 1986; **7**: 916–24.

[2] Hearse DJ, Yellon DM, Downey JM.
Can beta blockers limit infarct size?
Eur Heart J 1986; **7**: 925–30.

[3]   Reimer KA, Jennings RB, Cobb FR, *et al.*
      Animal models for protecting ischemic
      myocardium: results of the NHLBI
      Cooperative Study.
      Circ Res 1985; **56**: 651–65.

[4]   Hearse DJ.
      The protection of the ischemic myocardium:
      surgical success versus clinical failure?

FREE RADICALS AND THE PATHOPHYSIOLOGY OF TISSUE INJURY IN THE HEART DURING ISCHAEMIA AND REPERFUSION

D.J. HEARSE

Free radicals

A free radical is any intermediate that contains one or more unpaired electrons and is capable of independent existence [1]. The unpaired electrons render the molecule very reactive and short-lived. There are free radicals of many elements including carbon, nitrogen and sulphur, but this presentation will concentrate on the radicals of oxygen. Normally, molecular oxygen in the body is reduced to water, in a tetravalent manner, by the mitochondria. However, if oxygen is univalently reduced in a stepwise manner, we see the sequential formation of the superoxide radical, hydrogen peroxide and the hydroxyl radical. These three intermediates are all highly reactive and potentially toxic [2].

Free radicals are formed not only under pathological conditions but also in the course of normal metabolism and many sources of generation of radicals exist. Perhaps the best known source, particularly important during ischaemia and reperfusion, relates to the breakdown of ATP to adenosine and the movement of adenosine from the myocyte to the endothelium, where it is converted into xanthine. Through the action of the enzyme xanthine oxidase, it is then converted to uric acid using molecular oxygen as a substrate, generating superoxide and hydrogen peroxide as by-products [3]. Another important source of free radicals are the leukocytes, which are capable of generating large quantities of various radicals. Haemoglobin and myoglobin are other potentially important sources of radicals, particularly under hypoxic conditions. Mitochondria metabolize almost all of their oxygen via tetravalent pathways, but 1%-2% is processed via the univalent pathway such that mitochondria continually produce small quantities of superoxide and other radicals. The arachidonic acid pathway is another source of radicals, as indeed are catecholamines.

Pathophysiology of tissue injury

Being highly reactive, free radicals can cause many different kinds of damage within the myocardium, including lipid peroxidation, nucleic acid injury, inhibition of enzymes, ultrastructural damage and protein degradation.

The two best known effects of free radicals are lipid peroxidation and redox changes to carrier proteins. If a radical, such as a hydroxyl radical, is produced in the vicinity of the cell membrane, it can react with a polyunsaturated fatty acid which in the presence of oxygen can initiate a chain reaction leading to the production of many lipid peroxide molecules. This process will continue until terminated by either a radical-radical interaction or scavenging by some endogenous antioxidant, such as vitamin E.

The other well known aspect of radical-mediated injury is the alteration of the activity of membrane carrier proteins. For example, sodium-calcium exchange activity is thought to be controlled, in part, by a number of sulphydryl groups in the carrier protein molecule. In the presence of a variety of oxidant species, it is possible to oxidize these groups to form a disulfide bridge and hence alter the activity of the carrier. Similar changes are known for many other carrier proteins, such as sodium-potassium ATPase and calcium-magnesium ATPase. In this way, free radicals can dramatically alter ionic homeostasis.

Anti-oxidant enzymes

Over the course of evolution, sophisticated anti-oxidant defence mechanisms have been developed to deal with normal levels of radical production in the myocardium and other tissues. The best known of the so-called 'anti-oxidant enzymes' is superoxide dismutase, which converts (dismutates) superoxide radicals to hydrogen peroxide and oxygen. The enzyme catalase then breaks down the hydrogen peroxide to water, thus avoiding the formation of the particularly dangerous hydroxyl radical. In normal circumstances, these enzymes protect cells against the consequences of radical production. These defences are supplemented by large numbers of cellular anti-oxidants, strategically located within the cell. For instance, in lipid soluble compartments such as membranes, alpha tocopherol is present, while in the water soluble compartment of the cytoplasm, ascorbate is found.

What happens in the heart under pathological conditions? There have been several studies in the last ten years from which a very interesting concept has emerged. Namely, that myocardial ischaemia is thought to prime the myocardium such that, at the time of reperfusion, there is a sudden burst of radical production that overwhelms endogenous defence mechanisms and causes additional damage. Thus, ischaemia promotes leukocyte infiltration; reperfusion will bring more of these cells into the myocardium and they represent potent sources of radicals, particularly in damaged tissue. Mitochondrial metabolism is disrupted and there is a strong possibility that univalent reduction will increase and as a result more radicals will be produced. Ischaemia and reperfusion stimulate and promote catecholamine overflow and arachidonic acid metabolism, again sources of radical production. During ischaemia, there is a net degradation of adenine nucleotides to hypoxanthine and this builds up in the myocardium; it is suggested that ischaemia also promotes the conversion of xanthine dehydrogenase — the safe form of this enzyme — to its oxidase form. At the same time, as a consequence of ischaemia, there is a loss of superoxide dismutase activity and loss of organic anti-oxidants within the cell. All these factors combine to increase radical production, particularly at the time of reperfusion.

Radical production during reperfusion

Only very recently has definitive evidence been obtained to support the idea that radicals are formed in a 'burst' during the early moments of reperfusion. In a joint study with Professor T. Slater at Brunel University, we were one of the first groups to chart radical production in the heart using electron spin resonance spectroscopy — the only method which allows radical production to be directly measured [4]. In this particular study, hearts were subjected to 15 minutes of ischaemia and then reperfused; a transient but substantial burst of radical production was observed. Studies in the dog and a number of other species have confirmed that after relatively short periods of ischaemia (10-30 minutes duration) there appears to be a dramatic burst of radical production during the early moments of reperfusion.

Having established that radicals are indeed produced, consideration must now be given to their potential significance. At present, attention is focused on three areas. Firstly, there is the possibility that this burst of radicals, which may occur for five or ten minutes after reperfusion, may play a role in the genesis of reperfusion arrhythmias. Secondly, there is considerable interest that these radicals may contribute to the outcome of myocardial infarction, particularly where reperfusion is involved, and that radicals may also contribute very substantially to the phenomenon known as myocardial 'stunning'. Thirdly, in cardiac surgery and transplantation, where there is global ischaemia and reperfusion, there is now considerable evidence suggesting that radicals may play a role in determining the outcome of the reperfusion process. What evidence is available to support these propositions?

Reperfusion arrhythmias

With respect to reperfusion arrhythmias, there are now many studies in several species, both *in vivo* and *in vitro*, which show that a variety of rather diverse agents, all capable of inhibiting radical production or scavenging radicals once they are formed, have anti-arrhythmic properties. The theory has evolved that, during the early moments of reperfusion when the burst of radical production occurs, these radicals attack cell membranes, either by lipid peroxidation or by altering the redox state of ion pumps. This leads to changes in membrane permeability — specifically a loss of potassium and a gain of sodium and calcium — that will promote arrhythmo-genesis.

Is there any evidence to support this hypothesis? A great deal of research into this issue has been undertaken, most involving studies in the rat heart, *in vivo* and *in vitro*. After brief (5-15 minutes) periods of ischaemia followed by reperfusion, there is a very high incidence (80%-100%) of arrhythmias in this model. A wide range of anti-oxidants — superoxide dismutase, catalase, glutathione, methionine, desferal and mannitol — all produce similar, substantial, reductions in the incidence of reperfusion arrhythmias [5].

There is growing evidence to indicate that *enhancing* radical production *increases* the likelihood of arrhythmias developing. We have investigated this phenomenon, using the fluorescein derivative Rose Bengal. This compound can be photoactivated by green light and when this occurs in the presence of molecular oxygen, reactive oxygen intermediates (superoxide and singlet oxygen) are formed. Prior to its photoactivation Rose Bengal has no effect on the heart, and it is possible to perfuse isolated rat hearts with solutions containing this compound without changes in coronary flow, heart rate or inotropic state. If the heart is then illuminated to activate the Rose Bengal and generate a burst of oxidant stress, there is the rapid evolution of cardiac arrhythmias. We have conducted dose-response studies of this phenomenon and found it to be dependent on the dose of Rose Bengal (nanomolar amounts are effective) and the intensity of the illumination.

Outcome of myocardial infarction

Most studies concerned with the role of radicals in the evolution of myocardial infarction have been conducted in dogs. The use of anti-oxidants — superoxide dismutase, catalase, oxypurinol and dimethylthiourea — has been shown to cause marked reductions in the size of myocardial infarcts.

Myocardial 'stunning' is the term given to a prolonged, but reversible, post-ischaemic contractile depression that may follow a relatively brief period of ischaemia. There is now a convincing body of data indicating that free radical generation during the early moments of reperfusion is one of the primary causes of stunning. To this end it has been shown that the administration of anti-oxidants can dramatically attenuate stunning in dogs.

Outcome of cardiac surgery

Finally, in the field of cardiac surgery, several studies in animal hearts, including work in our laboratories with superoxide dismutase and catalase, have indicated that anti-oxidants can have beneficial effects during global ischaemia and reperfusion.

Conclusions

It would seem then that there is strong evidence to associate free radical formation with several of the most striking pathophysiological features of myocardial ischaemia and reperfusion. Doubts persist, however, and the importance of radicals in ischaemia (in the absence of reperfusion) remains controversial. We do not know precisely which radicals are important, nor can we explain how agents such as superoxide dismutase, that are confined to the plasma, are able to protect the cells of the myocardium. There is a growing interest in the use of anti-radical measures to reduce the risk of reperfusion arrhythmias — an application which may be relevant to thrombolysis — as a means of reducing ischaemic damage and as a protection against stunning in situations of infarction or cardiac surgery. Nevertheless, much work remains to be done before the place of such interventions in cardiology is finally established.

References

[1] Halliwell B, Gutteridge JMC.
    Free radicals in biology and medicine.
    Oxford Scientific Publications, 1985.
[2] Bulkley GB.
    The role of oxygen free radicals in human disease processes.
    Surgeon 1983; **94:** 407–11.
[3] Hearse DJ.
    Free radicals and myocardial injury during ischaemia and reperfusion: a short-lived phenomenon? In: M Rosen, ed. *Lethal arrhythmias resulting from myocardial ischaemia and infarction.* Boston: Kluwer, 1988; 105–15.

[4] Garlick PB, Davies MJ, Hearse DJ, Slater TF.
    Direct detection of free radicals in the reperfused heart using electron spin resonance spectroscopy.
    Circ Res 1987; **61:** 757–60.
[5] Bernier M, Hearse DJ, Manning AS.
    Reperfusion-induced arrhythmias and oxygen-induced free radicals: studies with anti-free radical interventions and a free radical generating system in the isolated perfused rat heart.
    Circ Res 1986; **58:** 331–340.

FATTY ACIDS, ARRHYTHMIAS AND MYOCARDIAL ISCHAEMIA

M.F. OLIVER

In considering the possible role of free fatty acids (FFA) in the genesis of arrhythmias, two questions need to be addressed. Are there situations when raised plasma FFA can be arrhythmogenic and, if so, are some fatty acids more likely to display this property than others?

Arrhythmogenic role of free fatty acids

In formulating the first proposition [1], we demonstrated [2,3] that ventricular arrhythmias were a more frequent complication of acute myocardial infarction when the FFA:albumin molar binding ratio was greater than 2; this corresponds approximately to FFA levels of 1200 µEq/l (Fig. 1). Not all subsequent studies confirmed this finding, but the balance of evidence from these later investigations sustained the conclusions of the original proposal. More recently, Tansey & Opie [4] have confirmed that high FFA levels are indeed associated with an increased incidence of ventricular arrhythmias during acute infarction.

We have previously described the relationship between FFA and myocardial function. Intravenous infusions of lipid-free albumin, e.g. a low FFA/albumin ratio, to dogs during acute coronary occlusion reduced the extent of myocardial ischaemia in contrast to control infusions with a normal FFA/albumin ratio [5]. Reduction of plasma FFA by beta-pyridylcarbinol also decreased the severity of myocardial injury

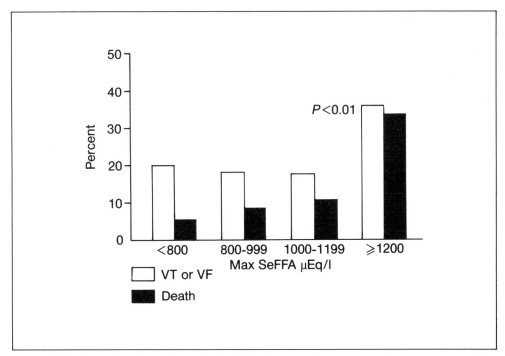

Fig. 1. Incidence of VT or VF, and deaths, in 200 consecutive patients with acute myocardial infarction.

[6]. Elevation of plasma FFA by infusions of intralipid and heparin during experimental coronary occlusion in dogs increased the incidence of ventricular arrhythmias [7].

Further persuasive support for an arrhythmogenic role for FFA comes from a study of patients with acute myocardial infarction in which it was possible to prevent excessive mobilization of FFA from peripheral tissues by administration of a nicotinic acid analogue [8]. When this treatment effectively prevented any increase in plasma FFA levels during the first two to five hours post-myocardial infarction, no incident of ventricular tachycardia or fibrillation developed in contrast to a high incidence in a comparable control group. This study has not been repeated — the particular drug can provoke histamine-mediated reactions and there were also problems with tachyphylaxis. It is important to know if other lipolytic agents are also able to prevent or eliminate arrhythmias, and it is surprising that this therapeutic possibility has not attracted more attention.

Identifying arrhythmogenic fatty acids

The first of our two questions having, essentially, been answered in the affirmative, more recently interest has been focused on the potential of individual fatty acids, particularly the polyunsaturated n-6 and n-3 fatty acids. The principal n-6 fatty acid is linoleic acid: it is an essential fatty acid and the precursor for the synthesis of arachidonic acid. The most familiar example of an n-3 fatty acid is eicosapentaenoic acid, present in fish oils.

Evidence has existed for several years to show that some patients with angina and acute infarction have low levels of adipose and platelet linoleic acid [9]. This inverse association between linoleic acid levels and angina/myocardial infarction is as strong, statistically, as the direct relation between total or LDL-cholesterol and coronary disease and is independent of it. The only confounding factor is a low intake of linoleic acid in smokers [10].

Feeding studies in rats have indicated that an increase in the proportion of dietary fat derived from n-6 polyunsaturates (hence increasing linoleic acid levels) is associated with a substantially reduced incidence of ventricular fibrillation during subsequent *in vitro* myocardial hypoxia [11]. About three months of increased polyunsaturate intake are required before this becomes apparent. Lepran *et al.* have studied this phenomenon in the more realistic setting of experimental coronary occlusion in rats, and have produced essentially similar results [12]. Australian investigators have demonstrated that pre-feeding of dogs with diets rich in n-3 fatty acids significantly reduced the incidence of ventricular arrhythmias during coronary artery infarction [13].

We have conducted similar studies and found that in rats fed on a diet with a polyunsaturated fat:saturated fat (P:S) ratio of 2:0, the incidence of ventricular fibrillation following coronary artery ligation is much lower than in rats fed a diet with a P:S ratio of 0:3 (Table 1) [14]. No parallel reduction in ventricular tachycardia occurred, but given the different mechanisms underlying fibrillation and tachycardia, there is no reason to assume that both would be affected in the same way. While these and similar studies show consistently that diets increasing linoleic acid levels reduce the incidence of arrhythmias, results from clinical studies are less emphatic.

Abraham *et al.* undertook a retrospective study of coronary care unit patients with documented ventricular arrhythmia to relate the incidence of arrhythmia to adipose tissue distribution of fatty acids [15]. There was a marginally significant excess of incidence of arrhythmias in patients with greater proportions of saturated fatty acids. There was only a non-significant trend towards lower levels of linoleic acid in patients

Table 1. Effect of different diets on ventricular arrhythmias in rats.

Diet	No.	VF	VT
40% cal P/S 0.3	37	65%	95%
40% cal P/S 2.0	35	34%	80%
30% cal P/S 0.3	39	77%	100%
30% cal P/S 2.0	39	31%	90%

with arrhythmias, a result at variance with the data from animal studies. Abraham subsequently undertook a prospective study of patients admitted with acute myocardial infarction (22 patients with ventricular arrhythmia and 84 patients who did not develop arrhythmia). Again, correlations between the incidence of arrhythmia, P:S ratio and individual fatty acids were weak, and of only marginal statistical significance (Table 2).

Faced with this contradiction in results between human and animal studies, we thought that it might be more appropriate to study platelet fatty acids, since a measure of the fatty acid composition of a mixture of platelet phospholipids would be obtained. Such a study was made in 16 patients with ventricular fibrillation (and 32 patients with acute infarction but without ventricular fibrillation) at the Cardiovascular Research Unit, University of Edinburgh. No differences in the levels of platelet saturated fatty acids, or of n-6 or n-3 fatty acids, were found.

This inability to replicate in patients the results of animal studies may indicate that pre-feeding studies in animals should not be expected to be replicated by cross-sectional surveys in patients. In this regard, a recent report is particularly interesting: in patients given advice to eat fish twice weekly after myocardial infarction, there was a lower mortality (but not morbidity) rate two years later [16]. This opens the question of whether patients with angina but no infarction might be protected from ventricular

Table 2. Mean percentage adipose tissue fatty acid composition of patients with and without ventricular fibrillation.

Sum of fatty acids	Retrospective study		Prospective study	
	VF (*n* = 7)	No VF (*n* = 35)	VF (*n* = 22)	No VF (*n* = 84)
Saturates	32.5**	29.7	32.1*	30.7
Monoenes	26.8*	28.1	26.9	27.6
Polyenes	10.0	10.6	10.4	10.3
n-6	9.7	10.4	10.2	10.0
n-3	0.3	0.3	0.2	0.3
P/S ratio	0.31*	0.36	0.33	0.34

Mann Whitney U Test: *$P<0.05$; **$P<0.01$

arrhythmias by adjusting their diets in order to increase the P:S ratio of plasma and myocardial fatty acids.

Conclusion

There is sufficient experimental data to support the proposition that polyunsaturated fatty acids influence the development of arrhythmias, but more detailed investigations will be required to establish this in humans. As to the mechanisms of this effect, there are several possible avenues: increased platelet aggregation; adverse effects on anti-oxidant systems; and altered esterification of individual phospholipids may make cells more vulnerable to the actions of free radicals or affect the ion transfer systems that operate in cell membranes. Any or all of these changes, plus others as yet unappreciated, may increase the risk of arrhythmias developing when the proportions of n-6 and n-3 acids are low.

How strong or clinically relevant is the relationship between individual fatty acids and arrhythmia, and whether or not fatty acid deficiency is an independent risk factor for arrhythmia in humans, are questions that still await resolution.

References

[1] Kurien VA, Oliver MF.
A metabolic cause for arrhythmias during acute myocardial hypoxia.
Lancet 1970; **i:** 813–5.

[2] Oliver MF, Kurien VA, Greenwood TW.
Relation between serum-free fatty acids and arrhythmias and death after acute myocardial infarction.
Lancet 1968; **i:** 710–5.

[3] Kurien VA, Yates PA, Oliver MF.
The role of free fatty acids in the production of ventricular arrhythmias after acute coronary artery occlusion.
Eur J Clin Invest 1971; **1:** 225–41.

[4] Tansey MJB, Opie LH.
Relation between plasma free fatty acids and arrhythmias within the first 12 hours of acute myocardial infarction.
Lancet 1983; **ii:** 419–22.

[5] Miller NE, Mjos OD, Oliver MF.
Relationship of epicardial ST segment elevation to the plasma free fatty acid/albumin ratio during occlusion in dogs.
Clin Sci Mol Med 1976; **51:** 209–13.

[6] Kjekhus JK, Mjos OD.
Effect of inhibition of lipolysis on infarct size following experimental coronary artery occlusion.
J Clin Invest 1973; **52:** 1770–8.

[7] Kurien VA, Yates PA, Oliver MF.
The role of free fatty acids in the production of ventricular arrhythmias after acute coronary artery occlusion.
Eur J Clin Invest 1971; **1:** 225–41.

[8] Rowe MJ, Neilson JMM, Oliver MF.
Control of ventricular arrhythmias during myocardial infarction by antilipolytic treatment using a nicotinic acid analogue.
Lancet 1975; **i:** 295.

[9] Wood DA, Riemersma RA, Butler S, *et al.*
Linoleic and eicosapentaenoic acids in adipose tissue and platelets and risk of coronary heart disease.
Lancet 1987; **i:** 177–83.

[10] Oliver MF.
Cigarette smoking, polyunsaturated fats, linoleic acid and coronary heart disease.
Lancet 1989; **i:** 1241–3.

[11] Saman S, Riemersma RA.
Dietary polyunsaturated fats reduce ischaemia induced ventricular fibrillation in the Langendorff perfused rat heart.
[Abstract]
Eur J Clin Invest 1985; **20:** A15.

[12] Lepran I, Nemecz G, Koltai M, Szekeres L.
Effects of a linoleic acid diet on the acute phase of coronary occlusion in conscious rats: influence of indomethacin and aspirin.
J Cardiovasc Pharmacol 1981; **3:** 847–53.

[13] McLennan PL, Abeywardena MY, Charnock JS.
Influences of dietary lipids on arrhythmias and infarctions after coronary ligation in rats.
Can J Physiol Pharmacol 1985; **63:** 1411–7.

[14] Riermersma RA, Sargent CA, Saman S, Rebergen SA, Abraham R.
Dietary fatty acids and ischaemic arrhythmias.
Lancet 1988; **i:** 285–6.

[15] Abraham R, Riemersma RA, Wood D, Elton R, Oliver MF.
Adipose fatty acid composition and the risk of serious ventricular arrhythmias in patients with acute myocardial infarct.
Am J Cardiol 1989; **63:** 269–72.

[16] Burr ML, Gilbert JF, Holliday RM, *et al.*
Effects of changes in fat, fish and fibre intakes on death and myocardial reinfarction: Diet and Reinfarction Trial (DART).
Lancet 1989; **ii:** 7.

INFARCT EXTENSION AND EXPANSION

R.M. NORRIS

Infarct extension

It is well established that infarction advances as a wave-front from endocardium to epicardium and that this process can be halted by thrombolysis — the earlier, the better. Given early thrombolysis and successful recanalization, infarct extension arises as a result of reocclusion of the infarct-related artery or, less commonly, from occlusion of another artery. Thus 'infarct extension' is really reinfarction by reocclusion of the infarct-related artery.

Recent data from the Auckland group of hospitals come from 456 patients who had thrombolysis (mean age 58 years) [1]. Most of the patients were participating in clinical trials of thrombolysis; 315 received streptokinase, 141 t-PA. Reinfarction was defined by the usual criteria — chest pain, enzyme changes, ST elevation and Q-waves. The overall 30-day incidence of reinfarction was 6%; the incidence was slightly higher with t-PA than with streptokinase, but not significantly so. At one-year follow-up, the reinfarction rate had risen to 9%. Eighty-six percent of these infarcts were in the same territory as the original infarct. Presumably the infarct-related artery that had been reperfused subsequently reoccluded.

Patients who had reinfarcted were compared with those who did not reinfarct, using coronary arteriography and left ventriculography. An interesting finding was that left ventricular function of the people who had reinfarction was only slightly more impaired than in those who had not had reinfarction [ejection fraction ($\pm$ SEM) $55 \pm 2\%$ *vs* $57 \pm 1\%$; end-systolic volume 68 ± 5 ml *vs* 65 ± 2 ml]. The mortality rate following reinfarction was 12%, so that if reinfarction occurred in 9% of cases, the total mortality rate from reinfarction of all the patients over one year was about 1%. This bears on Dr Fuster's comments (see page 12) about the severity of stenosis and the propensity to promote development of coronary collaterals — a tight stenosis is more likely to reocclude than a relatively mild one, but a patient with a tight stenosis may well have better collateral blood supply. So infarct extension with thrombolysis is a significant problem, but not the major one.

Infarct expansion

Infarct expansion is more important. The mechanism of infarct expansion has been elegantly studied in the rat heart by Weisman and colleagues from the Johns Hopkins

University [2]. A synopsis of their results is shown in Fig. 1. When the left coronary artery in the rat is tied off, a mainly free wall infarct results. The heart may be sectioned and graphs plotted to show wall thickness and number of cells in the different areas of the heart (Fig. 1). Three very important points emerge from this analysis. The first is that the major infarct expansion occurred on day one; not very much more occurred on days two and three. The second is that thinning of the wall occurred in the normal zone and not just in the infarct zone. Point three is that there was a very close correlation between thinning of the wall and the number of cells counted in the wall, so that the mechanism of thinning seemed to be cell slippage rather than stretching of cells. These workers were able to show the same event in human hearts.

McKay, Grossmann and colleagues [3] published an important paper in 1986 examining infarct expansion and remodelling. Fig. 2 shows ventriculograms from this study taken from two patients at 10 hours after the onset of infarction, and again at two weeks. Not only was the area of the infarct greater at two weeks than at 10 days, but also the normal zone had expanded between 10 days and two weeks. On the basis of this and related studies, these workers developed what is perhaps the best theory of ventricular remodelling. They proposed that lengthening of the endocardial

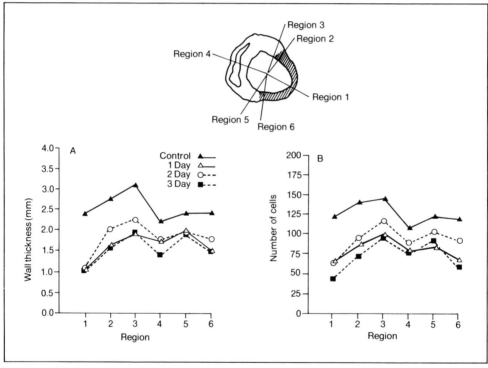

Fig. 1. This is a composite diagram taken from a publication by Weisman and colleagues [2] describing mechanisms of infarct expansion in the rat heart. Regions of the left ventricular infarct which were sampled are shown at the top, the wall thickness of regions compared with control hearts at 1, 2 and 3 days after coronary artery ligation at bottom left, and the number of cells comprising the wall thickness at bottom right. Data show that (1) most of the wall thinning has occurred by Day 1; (2) non-infarcted regions (regions 3 and 5) undergo wall thinning as well as the infarcted regions (1, 2 and 6); (3) reduction in cell numbers in the wall parallels reduction in wall thickness. (Reproduced with permission from Weisman HF, Bush DE, Mannise JA, *et al. Circulation* 1988; **78:** 186–201. [2])

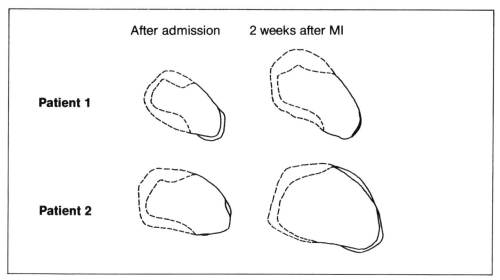

Fig. 2. Right anterior oblique end-diastolic and end-systolic cardiac silhouettes in 2 patients after admission (left) and at two weeks (right) after myocardial infarction. Solid lines indicate infarcted segments and stippled lines indicate non-infarcted areas. In both cases there has been an increase in chamber volume as well as lengthening of both the infarcted and non-infarcted perimeters. (Reproduced with permission from McKay RG, Pfeffer MA, Pasternak RC, *et al. Circulation* 1986; **74**: 693–702. [3])

perimeter without regional wall motion abnormalities and with no evidence of wall thinning, suggested the occurrence of volume overload hypertrophy in diastole. Such volume overload hypertrophy implies an increase in myocardial mass, that is remodelling, by series addition of new sarcomeres and fibre elongation. By contrast, in pressure overload, hypertrophy is concentric by addition of new sarcomeres in parallel.

Measurement of infarct expansion
How should infarct expansion be measured? Traditionally left ventricular function is described in terms of ejection fraction, but ejection fraction is merely an arithmetic term and if we are looking at expansion we should be using volumes. At Green Lane Hospital, a study has been undertaken in a large series of patients ($n = 605$) who have been studied for many years with a mean follow-up of 6.5 years [4]. These were patients with first and second myocardial infarctions, with angiocardiography performed one to two months after the event. We looked for prognostic factors from the angiocardiogram, and on univariate analysis by the log rank test it was found that end-systolic volume was considerably the most powerful. End-systolic volume was better than end-diastolic volume in predicting mortality; end-diastolic volume, in turn, was better than ejection fraction. Myocardial score, which reflected the severity of coronary disease, was further down the list, and other factors were of still less importance. Applying the proportional hazards model, it was found that prognosis could be completely described in terms of systolic volume and the square of systolic volume, implying that the relationship between systolic volume and risk was curvilinear rather than linear (Fig. 3). The only other independent prognostic indicator was continued cigarette smoking.

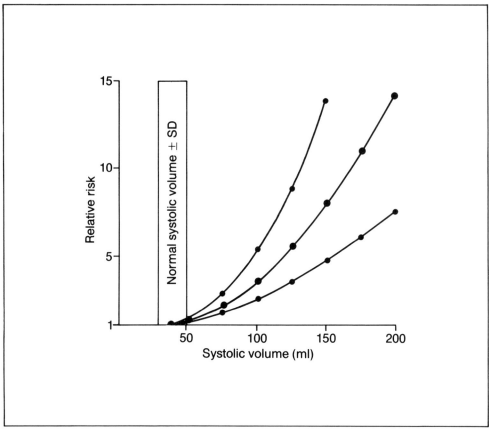

Fig. 3. Curve of relative risk of cardiac death ($\pm$ 95% confidence limits) versus end-systolic volume after recovery from myocardial infarction. Risk does not increase markedly until end-systolic volume is raised by 3-4 SD's above normal, but thereafter rises steeply. (Reproduced with permission from White HD, Norris RM, Brown MA, *et al. Circulation* 1987; **76:** 44–51. [4])

Why is end-systolic volume rather than end-diastolic volume the important variable to measure? The answer emerges from a consideration of Fig. 4. This shows data from 53 patients with atypical chest pain and normal coronary arteries, 80 myocardial infarction victims who had not had thrombolysis, and 312 infarction victims who had had thrombolysis. One month post-myocardial infarction, end-systolic volume in the second group was 87% greater than in the patients with normal coronary arteries. In patients treated with thrombolysis, it is 56% greater. In both groups, however, end-diastolic volume has increased by only 9%–17%.

McKay, Grossmann, *et al.* [3] have also studied infarct expansion, measuring end-systolic and end-diastolic volumes, plus ejection fraction, in a group of patients 10 hours and 14 days after infarction. These patients all had successful thrombolysis. Increases in end-systolic and end-diastolic volumes were observed between 10 hours and 14 days, while ejection fraction was preserved (Fig. 5). At two weeks, left ventricular end-diastolic pressure was lower and cardiac index slightly higher than immediately post-infarction. Evidently, myocardial remodelling had occurred, leading to maintenance of ejection fraction at the expense of ventricular dilatation. Previous findings from normal subjects in these workers' laboratory [5] support our finding that end-systolic volume increases by around 100% after infarction, whereas end-diastolic volume increases by only about 20%.

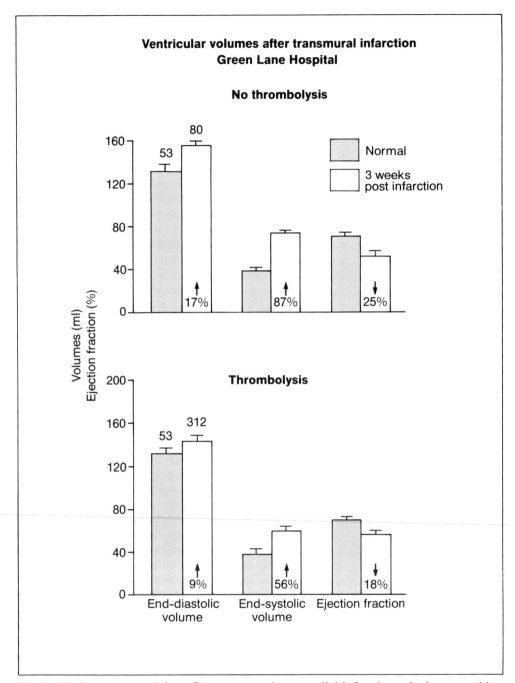

Fig. 4. Patients recovered from first transmural myocardial infarction, whether treated by thrombolysis or not, differ from normal subjects mainly by an increase in left ventricular end-systolic volume. See text for details.

Prevention of infarct expansion

Clearly, the processes of infarct expansion and ventricular remodelling, as reflected by end-systolic volume, are significant adverse prognostic factors. What can be done to prevent infarct expansion? Sharpe [6] and Pfeffer [7] have recently published

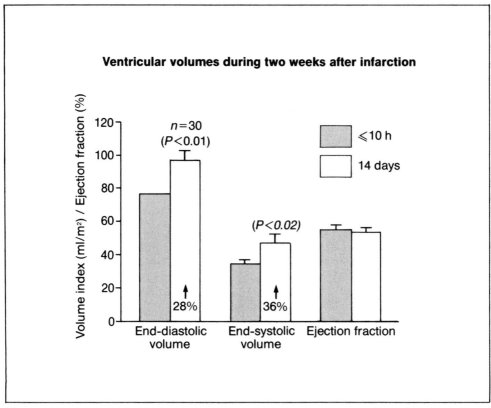

Fig. 5. Increase in ventricular volumes between admission and ten days after admission for myocardial infarction treated by thrombolysis. Data from McKay *et al.* [3].

separate reports on the use of captopril to reduce afterload on the ventricle during the period of myocardial healing, post-myocardial infarction. Sharpe reported significantly lower end-systolic volumes in patients treated with captopril, and a significantly better ejection fraction. However, these patients were selected on the basis of an ejection fraction <45%; moreover, volumes were measured by echocardiography. Pfeffer et al. used ventriculography and revealed no overall benefit of captopril. It was shown that patients with blocked infarct-related arteries (about two-thirds of patients) did have better ventricular volumes after captopril, but this only emerged on retrospective analysis and was not apparent from the raw data. Again, these patients all had an ejection fraction <45%.

The weakness of both trials was the time of administration of captopril — Sharpe started treating his patients on day nine post-myocardial infarction, Pfeffer started on day 18. Referring to the experimental [2] and clinical [3] data, it seems likely that most of the infarct expansion had already occurred.

There is increasing evidence that a patent infarct-related artery at completion of myocardial necrosis has a favourable effect on limitation of infarct expansion. Trials of thrombolysis have focused on early (90-minute) patency, for which t-PA is clearly superior to streptokinase. When considering patency at 24 hours and three weeks, however, the two agents may be more comparable [8–10]. Thrombolysis for patients presenting later than four to six hours after symptom onset may be beneficial. Ways should be sought to enhance the efficacy of thrombolysis. Angioplasty appears to be unsuitable for this, but greater consideration should be given to anti-platelet agents, of which aspirin is only one of a number of possibilities.

Conclusion

Infarct expansion caused by cell slippage, with consequent dilatation and ventricular remodelling, is probably, in the setting of early effective thrombolysis, a more serious pathologic mechanism than infarct extension. Expansion is best quantified by end-systolic volume. Efforts to prevent expansion by reduction of ventricular wall stress may be possible. Thrombolysis may have a role to play in infarct expansion which is almost as important as its role in prevention of infarct extension. Expansion occurs early in the post-infarction phase and efforts to limit it should be initiated within the first 24 hours post-myocardial infarction.

References

[1] Rivers JT, White HD, Cross DB, *et al.*
Reinfarction after thrombolytic therapy
followed by conservative management:
incidence and effect of smoking.
J Am Coll Cardiol. In press.

[2] Weisman HF, Bush DE, Mannise JA, *et al.*
Cellular mechanisms of myocardial infarct
expansion.
Circulation 1988; **78**: 186-201.

[3] McKay RG, Pfeffer MA, Pasternak RC, *et al.*
Left ventricular remodelling after
myocardial infarction: corollary to infarct
expansion.
Circulation 1986; **74**: 693-702.

[4] White HD, Norris RM, Brown MA, *et al.*
Left ventricular end-systolic volume as the
major determinant of survival after recovery
from myocardial infarction.
Circulation 1987; **76**: 44-51.

[5] Wynne J, Green LH, Mann T, *et al.*
Estimation of ventricular volumes in man
from biplane cineangiograms filmed in
oblique projections.
Am J Cardiol 1978; **41**: 726.

[6] Sharpe N, Smith H, Murphy J, Hannon S.
Treatment of patients with symptomless left
ventricular dysfunction after myocardial
infarction.
Lancet 1988; **i**: 255-9.

[7] Pfeffer MA, Lamas GA, Vaughan DE, *et al.*
Effect of captopril on progressive left
ventricular dilatation after anterior
myocardial infarction.
N Engl J Med 1988; **319**: 80-6.

[8] The Thrombolysis in Myocardial Infarction
(TIMI) Study Group. Special Report.
The thrombolysis in myocardial infarction
(TIMI) trial. Phase I findings.
N Engl J Med 1985; **312**: 932-6.

[9] White HD, Rivers JT, Maslowski AH, *et al.*
Effect of intravenous streptokinase as
compared with that of tissue plasminogen
activator on left ventricular function after
first myocardial infarction.
N Engl J Med 1989; **320**: 817-21.

[10] PRIMI Trial Study Group.
Randomised double-blind trial of
recombinant pro-urokinase against
streptokinase in acute myocardial infarction.
Lancet 1989; **i**: 863-8.

3. THROMBOLYSIS

AN OVERVIEW OF THE EFFECTS OF DIFFERENT THROMBOLYTIC AGENTS ON MORTALITY AND ON MORBIDITY

R. COLLINS

Streptokinase is the most extensively studied fibrinolytic agent. Already more than 30,000 patients with suspected acute myocardial infarction have been randomized in trials comparing rapid high-dose (1.5 MU within one hour) intravenous streptokinase regimens with controls. Taken together [1,2] the results from all of these studies demonstrate clearly that streptokinase reduces mortality, and that the effects are greatest among patients treated most promptly — although there is evidence of some benefit even among those treated up to 24 hours from pain onset (reduction in odds of death at 0-3, 4-6 and 7-24 hours: 31% ± 5%, 22% ± 6% and 14% ± 6%, respectively). Newer fibrinolytic agents, such as t-PA and APSAC, may lyse coronary artery thrombi more effectively than intravenous streptokinase. Recently both t-PA [3] and APSAC [4] have been demonstrated to reduce mortality, compared with placebo, in patients presenting early (that is, within six hours of pain onset). No large direct comparisons between streptokinase, t-PA and APSAC are yet available, however, and so it is not yet known which fibrinolytic agent, if any, is most effective at averting cardiac death. GISSI-2 and ISIS-3, which involve direct large-scale randomized comparisons between different fibrinolytic agents, should help to resolve this issue.

When deciding whether to use fibrinolytic therapy in patients with suspected acute myocardial infarction, particularly those presenting late, it is necessary to consider not only the possible benefits but also the possible risks. Side-effects such as hypotension, allergic reactions (seen with streptokinase and APSAC) and minor bleeding (seen with all fibrinolytic agents) may be worrying but do not usually cause patients managed in hospital any serious problem. The recent trials [1-4] have demonstrated that the serious side-effects of fibrinolytic agents are rare (perhaps a few bleeds requiring transfusion and a few cerebral haemorrhages per 1000 patients, with no significant increase in the total number of strokes). On the other hand, the risk of coronary death in patients with suspected acute myocardial infarction may be high, even among those without pronounced ST elevation on their ECG or among those admitted later after symptom onset. A reduction in mortality of 'only' 14%, as suggested by the trial results for those presenting after six hours, would typically avoid about 15-20 early deaths among every 1000 patients, which compares favourably with the small number of serious complications that might be expected.

Review of all the fibrinolytic trials [1-4] does not support the suggestion [2] that the benefit among those treated within the first hour is much greater than among those treated slightly later, but a small decrease in the median time of treatment (for example, from five hours to four hours) [5] may produce a small improvement in the mortality reduction (for example, from 20% to 23%). Worthwhile improvements might therefore be achieved by simple measures, such as encouragement of prompt hospital admission and starting treatment in the emergency room before transfer to coronary care. However, it might be best to delay fibrinolytic treatment until hospital admission unless the patient's condition can be monitored during and after infusion, for there are side-effects (such as sudden profound hypotension and bleeding) that, although generally easy to manage in hospital, do require prompt medical attention. The safety and feasibility of pre-hospital use of fibrinolytic therapy is currently being evaluated [5].

In the ISIS-2 trial [1], aspirin was also found to reduce mortality by about one-fifth when used in acute myocardial infarction. The benefits of fibrinolytic therapy and of aspirin appeared to be largely independent of each other — that is, strep-tokinase reduced mortality by a roughly similar additional amount irrespective of whether aspirin was used or not, and vice versa (Fig. 1). The combination of both agents appeared to have serious side-effects that were no more frequent than those of streptokinase alone, yet the combination reduced the risk of disabling or fatal stroke and of reinfarction, as well as reducing mortality much more substantially than either agent does alone. For patients admitted early (that is, within six hours) the combination seemed to reduce mortality by about one-half, and even when used after a delay of several hours it seemed to reduce mortality by about one-third.

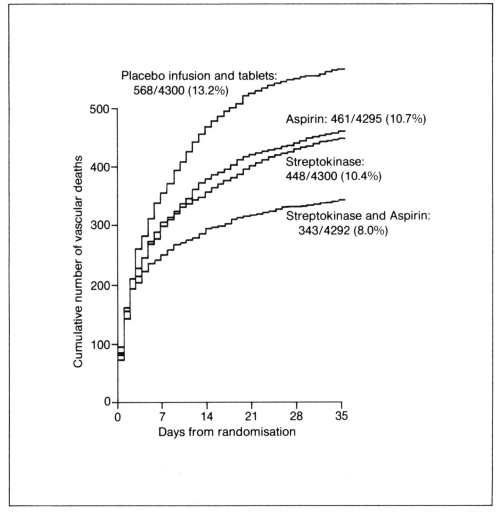

Fig. 1. Cumulative vascular mortality in days 0-35. (Reproduced with permission from ISIS-2 Collaborative Group, *Lancet* 1988; **ii:** 349–60. [1])

Aspirin does not require particularly careful monitoring, and it might well be appropriate to start it as soon as possible (in the home, ambulance or emergency room) provided there are no clear contraindications. Short-term anti-platelet therapy is likely to be applicable to almost all patients with suspected myocardial infarction, since the side-effects of low-dose aspirin seem negligible and the drug costs are small. Aspirin could be used widely not only in developed countries but also in countries with limited medical resources. If one month of low-dose aspirin were to be given to just one million new patients a year — which is only a fraction of the worldwide total with acute myocardial infarction — then a few tens of thousands of deaths, reinfarctions and strokes could be avoided or substantially delayed (and these benefits could be doubled if low-dose aspirin were continued for at least a few more years) [6] (Fig. 2).

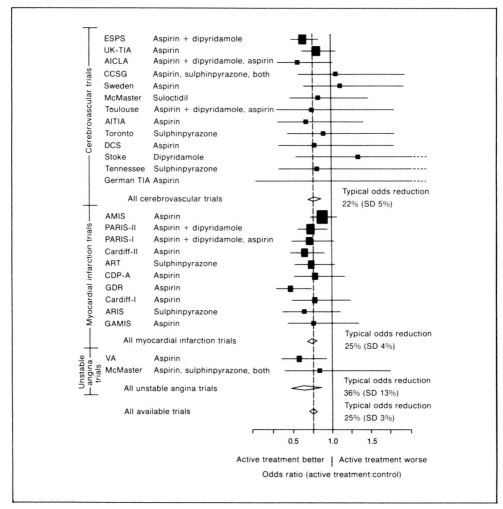

Fig. 2. Odds ratios (active treatment:control) for first stroke, myocardial infarction, or vascular death during scheduled treatment period in completed antiplatelet trials. —■— = Trial results and 99% confidence intervals (area of ■ proportional to amount of information contributed). ◇ = Overview results and 95% confidence intervals. Dashed vertical line represents odds ratio of 0.75 suggested by overview of all trial results. Solid vertical line represents odds ratio of unity (no treatment effect). (Reproduced with permission from Antiplatelet Trialists' Collaboration. *Br Med J* 1988; **296:** 320–31. [6])

Although further research may eventually identify some fibrinolytic or anti-thrombotic regimens more effective than streptokinase and aspirin, these agents are practicable and are of demonstrated value and safety. If both are used widely then they should avoid several tens of thousands of deaths worldwide each year.

References

[1] ISIS-II (Second International Study of Infarct Survival) Collaborative Group. Randomised trial of intravenous streptokinase, oral aspirin, both, or neither among 17,187 cases of suspected acute myocardial infarction: ISIS-2. *Lancet* 1988; **ii**: 349–60.

[2] GISSI. Effectiveness of intravenous thrombolytic therapy in acute myocardial infarction. *Lancet* 1986; **i**: 397–402.

[3] ASSET Study Group. Trial of tissue plasminogen activator for mortality reduction in acute myocardial infarction. *Lancet* 1988; **ii**: 525–30.

[4] AIMS Trial Study Group. Effect of intravenous APSAC on mortality after acute myo-cardial infarction: preliminary report of a placebo-controlled clinical trial. *Lancet* 1988; **i**: 545–9.

[5] European Myocardial Infarction Project (EMIP) Sub-committee. Potential time saving with pre-hospital intervention in acute myocardial infarction. *Eur Heart J* 1988; **9**: 118–24.

[6] Antiplatelet Trialists' Collaboration. Secondary prevention of vascular disease by prolonged antiplatelet treatment. *Br Med J* 1988; **296**: 320–31.

IMPORTANCE OF TIME WINDOW IN THROMBOLYTIC TREATMENT

R. SCHRÖDER

Introduction

In the ISAM study, 1741 patients were randomly allocated to either streptokinase or placebo. Infarct size was measured by the serum enzyme activity curve, cumulative release of MBCK and by the relative R-wave loss from the pre-randomization ECG to the ECG three weeks later [1]. One prospectively established aim of the study was that data from patients treated within three hours should be compared with data from those treated between three and six hours. Comparison showed that patients treated with streptokinase within three hours had significantly smaller infarcts than those treated later (Fig. 1). Analysis at hourly intervals revealed benefits in favour of strep-tokinase up to four hours, though this was really striking only in those patients treated within the first hour after symptom onset (Fig. 2). Similar results emerged from assessment of infarct size by ECG. In patients with inferior myocardial infarction, there were also significant differences between those treated within three hours; these differences stemmed mainly from those treated within the first two hours after symptom onset.

All these data would suggest that there is a time-window for salvage of ischaemic myocardium. The simplest way to shorten the interval between onset of symptoms and treatment, thereby bringing people within this window, is to initiate therapy outside hospital.

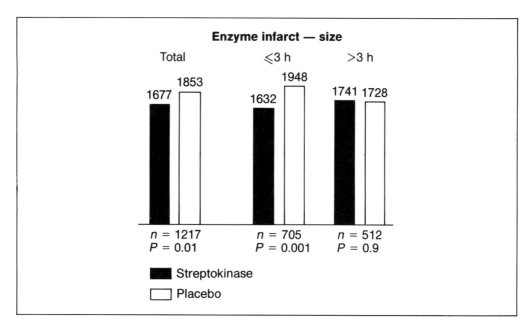

Fig. 1. Effect of early treatment with streptokinase on the area below the CK-MB serum time-activity curve.

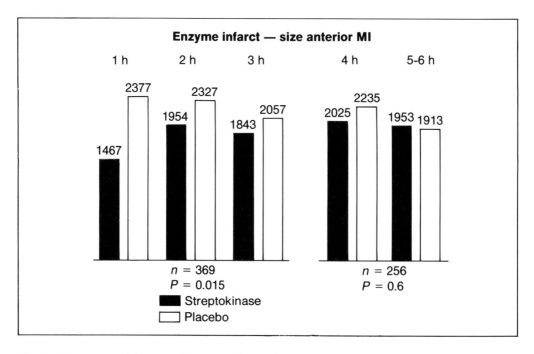

Fig. 2. Treatment with streptokinase conferred some benefit to patients with anterior myocardial infarction even when administered up to four hours after symptom onset.

This raises several questions and some years ago we performed controlled trials to answer a few of them. Specifically, is it safe for an experienced physician to conduct out-of-hospital thrombolysis, and is there actually a worthwhile time gain, even in a city like Berlin where there is a large network of mobile coronary care units and journey times to hospital are short [2]?

Experience has proved that the treatment is safe. Time savings are illustrated in Fig. 3, and are such that it is now regarded as routine in Berlin for mobile coronary care units to start thrombolytic therapy outside hospital.

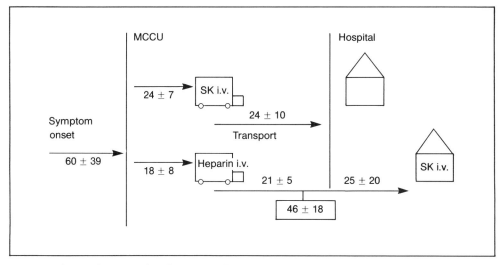

Fig. 3. Time gains resulting from out-of-hospital thrombolysis. Numbers represent minutes from symptom onset to arrival of the mobile coronary care unit (MCCU), until streptokinase or heparin was given randomly outside hospital, and until streptokinase was given in hospital to the latter group.

Patency of the infarct-related artery

Preliminary data (n=55) are available from a prospective investigation using 30 mg APSAC. Data on infarct size (estimated from enzyme release) endorsed the findings of the ISAM study, infarct size being substantially smaller (about 40%) in those treated within one hour compared to those treated between the second and third hour following onset of symptoms. Angiography was performed on these patients 10 days later and revealed a patency rate of 78%; in 70% of all there was TIMI grade 3 flow (that is, free run-off of contrast material). Left ventricular function 10 days post-infarction was similar in patients treated one, two or three hours after onset of symptoms. At first sight this seems surprising, but there is in fact a growing body of evidence that function some days after infarction is mainly determined by vessel patency, not infarct size. When the data were evaluated according to whether the infarcted arteries were patent or occluded, a significant difference in favour of patients with patent arteries was apparent even in this small cohort (Fig. 4). Thus, average ejection fraction in patients with patent arteries was 61% (51% in patients with occluded arteries), while the area of dysynergic left ventricle in patients with patent arteries was 40% smaller than in patients with occluded vessels.

Analysis of ten trials of thrombolytic therapy for which patency data are available indicates that the variable benefits of thrombolytic therapy (in terms of parameters such as ejection fraction) may be associated with the variable patency of infarct-related vessels post-thrombolysis (Table 1, Fig. 5) [1,3-11]. These findings support the view that left ventricular function after acute myocardial infarction is mainly determined by the patency of the infarct-related vessels.

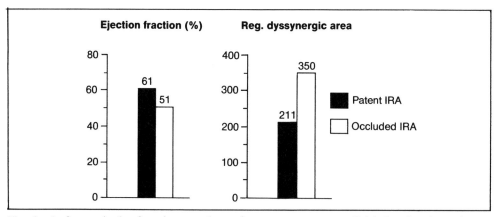

Fig. 4. Left ventricular function ten days after an acute myocardial infarction in patients with patent or occluded infarct-related arteries (IRA).

Table 1. Mode of death among patients receiving atenolol or control dying during days 0-1 of ISIS-I in UK, Ireland and Scandinavia only.

Reference			Ejection fraction %			Infarct artery patent %		
		Thrombolysis	Control	Differences in % ejection fractions	Thrombolysis	Control	Differences in % patency rates
O'Rourke	[3]	rt-PA	61	54	7	81	54	27
ICIN	[4]	i.c. SK	53	47	6	77	52	25
Australia	[5]	rt-PA	58	52	6	70	41	29
White	[6]	SK	59	53	6	75	54	21
APSIM	[7]	APSAC	53	47	6	77	36#	41 (day 4)
Armstrong	[8]	rt-PA	Adjustment for baseline differences		4	75	56	19
ISAM	[1]	SK	57	54	3	72	61#	11
ECSG	[9]	rt-PA	51	49	2	74	66#	8
Bassand	[10]	SK	45	44★	1	69	68	1
GEMT	[11]	APSAC	56	57	−1	75	76	−1

\# TIMI grade 3

★ radionuclide ventriculography

APSAC = anisoylated plasminogen streptokinase activator complex; i.c. = intracoronary; rt-PA = recombinant tissue plasminogen activator;

SK = streptokinase

Late patency of the affected artery

In order to ascertain if good vessel patency was beneficial if it occurred later in the course of myocardial infarction, we evaluated 368 patients from the ISAM study [12]. These patients were selected as having no early spontaneous or drug-induced reperfusion, on the basis of a late (that is, more than 15 hours after symptom onset) peak in their plasma CK-MB curves.

One month later 64% of patients who had been treated with streptokinase had a patent infarct-related artery, compared to 56% of those with therapeutic anticoagulation. The size of the acute infarcts was similar in patients with a patent or occluded artery. Indeed, infarct sizes as assessed by ECG and CK-MB were somewhat larger in the patients with patent arteries. Nonetheless, left ventricular function one month post-myocardial infarction was highly significantly better in those who had a patent

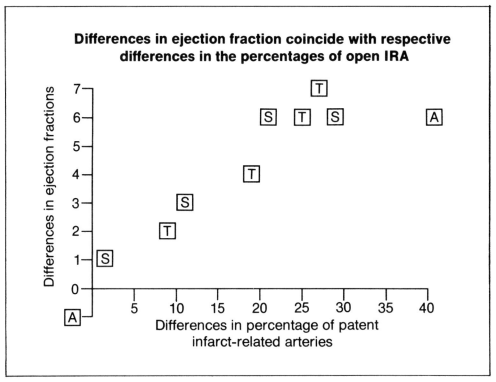

Fig. 5. Data from various thrombolysis trials at angiography 4-30 days after acute myocardial infarction. Differences in ejection fraction in favour of thrombolysis coincide with differences between patency rates of the infarct artery in thrombolysis and control groups. Each square refers to one trial. A = APSAC; S = streptokinase; T = tissue plasminogen activator (rt-PA). (Reproduced with permission from Schröder R, Neuhaus KL, Linderer T, *et al. Am J Cardiol* 1989; **64**: 878–84. [12])

artery as compared with those who had an occluded artery. There were similar significant differences with respect to disorders of regional wall motion. The largest differences in favour of the patent artery were seen in patients in whom the LAD was affected. Since left ventricular function at hospital discharge is the main predictor of long-term survival it might be expected that patency of an infarct-related LAD would also be an indicator of good long-term survival.

When patients were followed up for an average of 31 months, there was a 5% mortality rate in patients who had patent, infarct-related LAD vessels; mortality was 15% in patients with occluded LADs. Differences in mortality were most striking in patients with involvement of the proximal LAD (8% mortality when the vessel was patent; 28% when it was occluded). Differences in left ventricular function between occluded and patent vessels were also most pronounced in this group of patients (Fig. 6).

Conclusion
There is a time window for actual salvage of jeopardized ischaemic myocardium. This window is 'open' for about four hours after symptom onset and reduction in early in-hospital mortality probably is mainly related to intervention during that time. However, left ventricular function some days after myocardial infarction is mainly determined by the patency of the infarct-related artery, regardless of any degree of

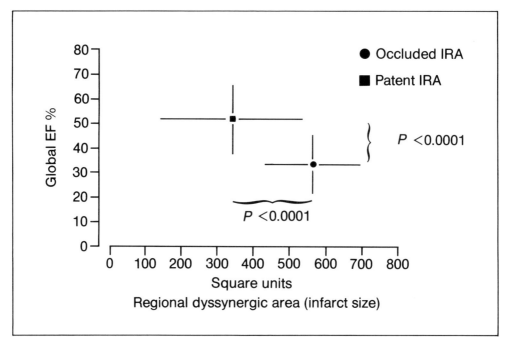

Fig. 6. Left ventricular function one month after myocardial infarction in 64 patients with proximal lesion of the LAD. (Reproduced with permission from Schröder R, Neuhaus KL, Linderer T, *et al. Am J Cardiol* 1989; **64:** 878–84. [12])

actual myocardial salvage. Thus, the effect of thrombolytic therapy on later in-hospital mortality and longer term survival may largely be due to its effect on the patency of infarct-related coronary arteries.

References

[1] ISAM Study Group.
A prospective trial of intravenous streptokinase in acute myocardial infarction (ISAM). Mortality, morbidity, and infarct size at 21 days.
N Engl J Med 1986; **314:** 1465–71.

[2] Bippus PH, Haux R, Schröder R.
Prehospital intravenous streptokinase in evolving myocardial infarction: a randomized study about feasibility, safety, and time-gain.
Eur Heart J 1987; **8**(suppl. 2):103.

[3] O'Rourke A, Baron D, Keogh A, *et al.*
Limitation of myocardial infarction by early infusion of recombinant tissue-type plasminogen activator.
Circulation 1988; **77:** 1311–5.

[4] Serruys PW, Suryapranata H, Simoons ML, *et al.*
Intracoronary thrombolysis in patients with acute myocardial infarction: The Netherlands Randomized Trial and current status.
Circulation 1987; **76-II:** 63–78.

[5] National Heart Foundation of Australia Coronary Thrombolysis Group.
Coronary thrombolysis and myocardial salvage by tissue plasminogen activator given up to 4 hours after onset of myocardial infarction.
Lancet 1988; **i:** 203–8.

[6] White HD, Norris RM, Brown AM, *et al.*
Effect of intravenous streptokinase on left ventricular function and early survival after acute myocardial infarction.
N Engl J Med 1987; **317:** 850–5.

[7] Bassand JP, Machecourt J, Cassagnes J, *et al.*
Multicenter trial of intravenous an..oylated plasminogen streptokinase activator complex (APSAC) in acute myocardial infarction: effects on infarct size and left ventricular function.
J Am Coll Cardiol 1989; **13:** 988–97.

[8] Armstrong PW, Baigrie RS, Daly PA, et al.
Tissue plasminogen activator: Toronto
(TPAT) placebo-controlled randomized trial
in acute myocardial infarction.
J Am Coll Cardiol 1989; **13:** 1469 76.

[9] Van der Werf F, Arnold A.
Intravenous tissue plasminogen activator
and size of infarct, left ventricular function,
and survival in acute myocardial infarction.
Br Med J 1988; **297:** 1374-9.

[10] Bassand JP, Faivre R, Becque O, et al.
Effects of early high-dose streptokinase
intravenously on left ventricular function in
acute myocardial infarction.
Am J Cardiol 1987; **60:** 435-9.

[11] Meinertz T, Kasper W, Schumacher M, Just
HJ, for the APSAC Multicenter Trial Group.
The German Multicenter Trial of
anisoylated plasminogen streptokinase
activator complex versus heparin for acute
myocardial infarction.
Am J Cardiol 1988; **62:** 347-51.

[12] Schröder R, Neuhaus KL, Linderer T, et al.
Impact of late coronary artery reperfusion of
left ventricular function one month after
acute myocardial infarction (Results from
the ISAM Study).
Am J Cardiol 1989; **64:** 878-84.

REPERFUSION RATES WITH DIFFERENT THROMBOLYTIC AGENTS

D. DE BONO

If the beneficial effect of coronary thrombolysis depends solely on the speed and efficacy of coronary reperfusion, then studies of angiographic reperfusion or patency rates are an effective way of comparing different thrombolytic regimes. The greatest precision will be achieved in studies which include pre-treatment angiography, but the delay in securing a pre-treatment angiogram may be to the patient's disadvantage, and because of clot 'ageing' the results might not mirror the clinical situation where thrombolytic therapy is given as promptly as possible. A more realistic compromise may be to compare patency at a set time, usually 90 minutes, after the start of treatment. Later assessments are unhelpful because of spontaneous reperfusion. It has to be emphasized that comparisons are of treatment regimes rather than individual drugs. Satisfactory dose ranging assessed by patency has only really been done for alteplase (rt-PA), and showed a positive relationship between dose and rate of reperfusion. However, clinical use of the highest dose (150 mg) was subsequently associated with unacceptable bleeding complications. A major problem is that much larger numbers of patients are needed for an accurate assessment of bleeding risk than of reperfusion rate. Data for streptokinase or anistreplase (APSAC) are more scanty, and it is probably wrong to assume that the dose response curve will resemble that for alteplase.

Within the limits of the technique, comparative studies of patency rates with different agents have shown a slight advantage of intravenous alteplase (70-100 mg) over streptokinase 1.5 million units. Patency rates with streptokinase 1.5 million units and anistreplase 30 mg are similar, but with a trend towards higher patency with anistreplase. Patency rates with alteplase 70 mg and urokinase 3 million units are similar. Heparin does not improve the patency rate over alteplase given alone. Data are not available on possible interactive effects of aspirin with thrombolytic agents on patency rates.

EFFECTS OF THROMBOLYSIS ON LEFT VENTRICULAR FUNCTION

R.M. NORRIS

Deterioration of left ventricular (LV) function is the most important adverse prognostic factor for patients after recovery from myocardial infarction. LV function is best described in terms of ejection fraction (EF) or end systolic volume (ESV). Clinical trials in which LV function has been measured have shown that early administration of thrombolytic drugs improves LV function in comparison with patients who have not received thrombolysis by between 25% and 33% towards normal; there is, however, no evidence that one drug is better than another for the preservation of LV function [1].

LV function as an end-point

If LV function is improved with thrombolysis, long-term survival should also be improved. Data from the Netherlands Inter-university trial [2] have shown that improved LV function after streptokinase administration has been reflected in a sustained reduction in mortality rates after hospital discharge.

LV function may then be used as a surrogate end-point for mortality [3]. This would be of great benefit in trials aiming to 'fine tune' the thrombolytic regimen, in terms of the number of patients who would have to be enrolled. To show a 20% reduction in mortality from a baseline of 5%, 15,000 patients would be required (two-sided α-error = 0.05; β-error = 0.2). Improvement of EF by a further 25% towards normal from a baseline of 59% by streptokinase treatment could be shown with 384 patients (same α- and β-errors) [3].

Results from a long-term study which we have carried out in Auckland have shown that ESV was superior to EF for the prediction of long-term survival in patients who did not receive thrombolytic therapy (Fig. 1) [4]. However, measurement of ESV has two disadvantages: it requires contrast ventriculography for accurate measurement and the range of values obtained is wider than for EF, necessitating greater trial numbers for equivalent statistical power.

The open infarct-related artery

There is some controversy about the infarct-related artery as a separate risk factor. Braunwald [5] proposes that late patency of the infarct-related artery is beneficial for three reasons. First, there is evidence that an opened infarct-related artery in the absence of thrombolysis gives better LV function. Second, in ISIS-II late reperfusion improved survival. Third, animal experiments show that late reperfusion promotes infarct healing.

However, clinical studies have produced conflicting evidence for this hypothesis. Between 1977 and 1984, patients presenting at Green Lane Hospital with transmural infarction received no thrombolytic agents. At four weeks after infarction, 75% of these patients had occluded infarct-related arteries. Outcome was better in the 25% of patients with patent infarct-related arteries who had higher EF and lower ESV than those who had occluded arteries [6]. Jeremy et al. in Sydney also showed that in patients who did not receive thrombolysis, LV function was better if the artery was open [7]. However in another study the increase in ventricular volume between 5 hours, 11 days and 10.5 months was no different in patients who had had successful

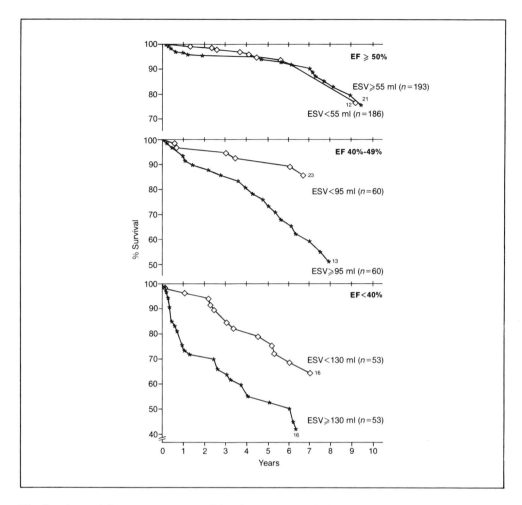

Fig. 1. Actuarial curves constructed for three groups of ejection fraction ($\geqslant 50\%$, 40%-49% and <40%), each group being subdivided according to whether end-systolic volume was above or below the median for that group. The greater predictive value of end-systolic volume is apparent only when ejection fraction is <50%. (Reproduced with permission from White HD, Norris RM, Brown MA, *et al. Circulation* 1987; **76:** 44–51. [4])

thrombolysis than in those who had not [8]. In a double-blind comparison of t-PA and streptokinase carried out in the Auckland group of hospitals, EF and ESV were the same with each treatment (Fig. 2) [9]. Whilst patients receiving t-PA almost certainly reperfused earlier [10], by three weeks after infarction patency rates with streptokinase were similar to those after t-PA. We do not know precisely when the 'late' reperfusion with streptokinase in our trial occurred, but it is likely that it occurred within 24 hours of treatment [11].

Conclusion
Thrombolysis improves LV function, improved LV function reduces late mortality and, therefore, LV function is an acceptable surrogate end-point for mortality. Patency of the infarct-related artery may be associated with improved LV function and hence improved survival, but not all the data are in agreement.

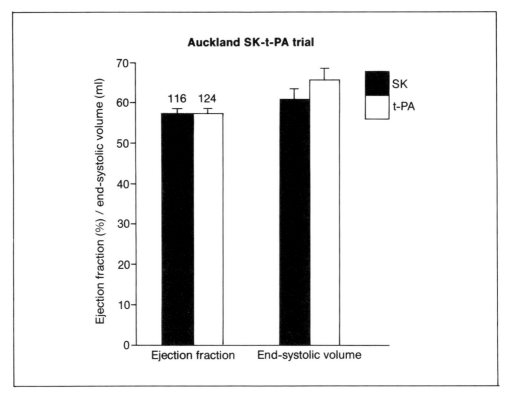

Fig. 2. Ejection fractions and end-systolic volumes found in a double-blind comparison of streptokinase with tissue plasminogen activator. (After White HD, Rivers JT, Maslowski AH, *et al. N Engl J Med* 1989; **320:** 817–21. [9])

References

[1]   Norris RM, White HD.
      Left ventricular function as an end point of
      thrombolytic therapy.
      Eur Heart Journal. Supplement. In press.

[2]   Simoons ML, Vermeer F, Vos J.
      Improved survival after thrombolytic
      therapy is maintained at five-year follow up.
      Circulation 1988; **78** (suppl.II): II–501.

[3]   Norris RM, White HD.
      Future therapeutic trials in coronary
      thrombosis should measure left ventricular
      function as the primary end-point of
      treatment.
      Lancet 1988; **i:** 104–6.

[4]   White HD, Norris RM, Brown MA, *et al.*
      Left ventricular end-systolic volume as the
      major determinant of survival after recovery
      from myocardial infarction.
      Circulation 1987; **76:** 44–51.

[5]   Braunwald E.
      Myocardial reperfusion, limitation of infarct
      size, reduction of left ventricular dysfunction
      and improved survival. Should the paradigm
      be expanded?
      Circulation 1989; **77:** 441–4.

[6]   Cross DB, White HD, Norris RM.
      The infarct-related coronary artery: late
      patency and left ventricular function with
      and without thrombolysis.
      Aust NZ J Med 1990; **20** (suppl.1): 341.

[7]   Jeremy RW, Hackworthy RA, Bautovich G,
      et al.
      Infarct artery perfusion and changes in left
      ventricular volume in the month after acute
      myocardial infarction.
      J Am Coll Cardiol 1987; **9:** 989–95.

[8]   Warren SE, Royal HD, Maskis JE, *et al.*
      Time course of left ventricular dilatation
      after myocardial infarction: influence of
      infarct-related artery and success of
      coronary thrombolysis.
      J Am Coll Cardiol 1988; **12:** 9–19.

[9]   White HD, Rivers JT, Maslowski AH, *et al.*
      Effect of intravenous streptokinase as
      compared with that of tissue plasminogen
      activator on left ventricular function after
      first myocardial infarction.
      N Engl J Med 1989; **320:** 817–21.

[11] PRIMI Trial Study Group. Randomised double-blind trial of recombinant pro-urokinase against streptokinase in acute myocardial infarction. *Lancet* 1989; **i:** 863–8.

[10] The Thrombolysis in Myocardial Infarction (TIMI) Study Group. Special Report. The thrombolysis in myocardial infarction (TIMI) trial. Phase I findings. *N Engl J Med* 1985; **312:** 932–6.

SPONTANEOUS REMODELLING OF CORONARY ARTERIES AFTER THROMBOLYSIS

M.E. BERTRAND

Prior to the era of thrombolytic treatment in acute myocardial infarction, De Wood *et al.* [1,2] showed that the incidence of coronary artery occlusion decreased significantly within the first 24 hours of myocardial infarction. Moreover, after two weeks only 53% of patients undergoing coronary angiography had complete coronary occlusion of the infarct-related vessel (Bertrand *et al.* [3]). These studies indicated that recanalization may occur spontaneously, without thrombolytic treatment.

Spontaneous recanalization after thrombolysis

When thrombolytic agents are administered, spontaneous recanalization may still occur. Rentrop *et al.* [4] assigned patients to intracoronary streptokinase or nitroglycerin. Patients receiving nitroglycerin showed a reduction in the incidence of coronary occlusion between one hour after myocardial infarction and 14 days. Where streptokinase failed to open the vessel, spontaneous recanalization was again observed in some patients at 14 days.

Even after apparently successful thrombolytic treatment, some residual narrowing of the infarct-related vessel may be found. Fig. 1 shows the extent of residual stenosis as measured at angiography immediately after administration of

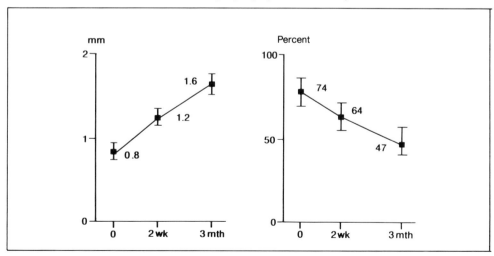

Fig. 1. Extent of residual stenosis immediately after administration of intracoronary streptokinase, two weeks and three weeks later. (Reproduced with permission from Cribier A, Saoudi N, Berland J, Letac B. *Arch Mal Coeur* 1985; **78:** 353. [5])

intracoronary streptokinase, and two weeks and three months later (Cribier *et al.* [5]). On the initial angiogram, there is a critical narrowing (75%) of the coronary artery. Two weeks later the narrowing is less critical, and after three months there is a non-significant narrowing at the site of the infarct-related vessel. Similar observations were made from data in the Western Washington trial.

Quantitative coronary angiography was performed to measure luminal diameter in three groups of patients (Brown *et al.* [6]). Evaluating the group of 13 patients with total coronary occlusion, there was a small decrease in the percentage of reduction of luminal diameter in the infarct-related vessel between initial examination at 30 minutes and repeat examination at 60 minutes and five weeks; some modification of the residual stenosis therefore seems likely. In five patients, coronary angiography was performed before myocardial infarction. There was a marked decrease in lumen diameter after infarction.

Using more sophisticated techniques of quantitative coronary angiography, Hackett *et al.* [7] studied residual stenosis immediately after administration of isosorbide dinitrate and one day later. There was a marked opening of the residual stenosis after infusion of the drug (Fig. 2).

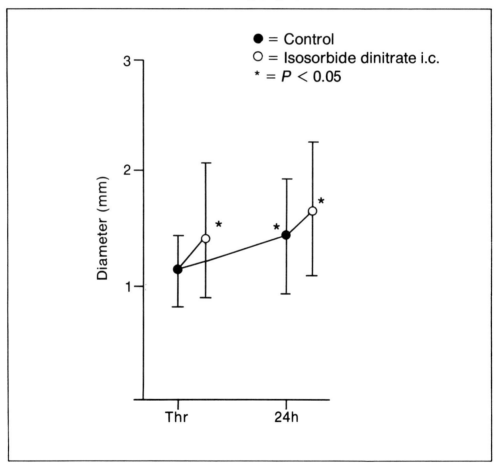

Fig. 2. Luminal diameter of the residual infarct-related stenoses at the end of thrombolysis (Thr), after intracoronary isosorbide dinitrate (ISDN) 2-4 mg, at 24 h, and after i.c. ISDN at 24 h. (Reproduced with permission from Hackett D, Davies G, Maseri A. *Eur Heart J* 1988; **9:** 1317–23. [7])

Mechanisms behind spontaneous remodelling

A number of hypotheses can be put forward to explain this 'remodelling' of coronary arteries. When the vessel is viewed immediately after administration of a thrombolytic agent, is thrombolysis incomplete and still continuing? Does the remodelling reflect some association between spontaneous recanalization and the thrombolytic agent? Thrombus forms both within the vessel lumen and inside the plaque. May there be some modification of the plaque? Vaso-constriction of the infarct-related vessel may affect its remodelling.

These observations on the spontaneous remodelling of coronary arteries after thrombolysis are not of academic interest alone, but have clinical implications. What are the long term consequences of remodelling, and should the time of thrombolytic treatment be extended? Also of importance is the appropriate timing for assessment of residual stenosis. This may have an impact on the perceived need for PTCA.

References

[1] DeWood MA, Spores J, Notske R, *et al.*
Prevalence of total coronary occlusion during the early hours of transmural myocardial infarction.
N Engl J Med 1980; **303**: 897–902.

[2] DeWood MA, Spores J, Hensley GR, *et al.*
Coronary arteriographic findings in acute transmural myocardial infarction.
Circulation 1983; **68** (suppl.1): 1–39, 1–49.

[3] Bertrand ME, Lefebvre JM, Laisne C, Rouseau M, Carre A, Lekieffre JP.
Coronary arteriography in acute myocardial infarction.
Am Heart J 1979; **97**: 61–9.

[4] Rentrop KP, Feit F, Blanke H, *et al.*
Effects of intracoronary streptokinase and intracoronary nitroglycerin infusion on coronary angiographic patterns and mortality in patients with acute myocardial infarction.
N Engl J Med 1984; **311**: 1457–63.

[5] Cribier A, Saoudi N, Berland J, Letac B.
Regression de la sténose coronaire résiduelle après recanalisation par fibrinolyse dans l'infarctus du myocarde. Analyse quantitative de la coronarographie immédiatement après désobstruction, au quinzième jour et au troisième mois de l'évolution.
Arch Mal Coeur 1985; **78**: 353.

[6] Brown BG, Gallery CA, Bagder RS, *et al.*
Incomplete lysis of thrombus in the moderate underlying atherosclerotic lesion during intracoronary infusion of streptokinase for acute myocardial infarction: quantitative angiographic observations.
Circulation 1986; **73**: 653.

[7] Hackett D, Davies G, Maseri A.
Pre-existing coronary stenoses in patients with first myocardial infarction are not necessarily severe.
Eur Heart J 1988; **9**: 1317–23.

NON-INVASIVE INDICES OF THROMBOLYSIS

W. KÜBLER

Early intravenous application of thrombolytic agents is nowadays recommended for the treatment of patients with acute myocardial infarction. The effectiveness of this form of therapy has been proven in two large randomized trials — GISSI and ISIS-II.

Footnote. This study was supported by a grant from the Deutsche Forschungsgemeinschaft, Bonn.

In an *individual* patient, however, the success or failure of intravenous thrombolysis is difficult to evaluate by non-invasive means. There are essentially four non-invasive methods which might be applied to the evaluation of reperfusion: clinical symptoms; the electrocardiogram (ECG); radioisotope cardiography; and measurement of marker proteins released from the infarcting area.

Symptoms
Immediately after successful thrombolysis, the patient generally feels some relief of anginal discomfort. This criteria is, however, purely subjective and depends greatly on the individual patient's sensitivity.

ECG
Apart from reperfusion arrhythmias, which are nonspecific and occur in variable degree, no other ECG signs exist which may be used as indicators for successful thrombolysis.

Radioisotope cardiography
This method is, in principle, a good way of demonstrating infarct reperfusion, especially if PET techniques can be employed. In practice, however, the time-consuming nature of the procedure makes it unsuitable for the evaluation of thrombolysis.

Marker proteins
Proteins are released from infarcting myocardium. Successful reperfusion leads to their more rapid release due to a more rapid washout from the infarcted tissue and induction of reperfusion injury. Four marker proteins were tested — creatine kinase (CK), CKMB (the CK isoform predominantly present in the myocardium), myoglobin, and myosin light chain.

Myoglobin is more rapidly released from the ischaemic myocardium than CK or CKMB. It is, however, not specific for myocardium; for instance, it exists in absolutely identical form in skeletal muscle. CKMB and myoglobin may be quantified by radioimmunoassays developed at the Heidelberg Clinic by Dr. Katus.

The same principles have been applied to the determination of myosin light chain. Myosin light chain is a structural protein of the myocardium; it has a specific structure which differs from that of myosin from smooth muscles or skeletal muscles. Myosin light chain is not normally present in plasma and hence offers certain advantages for the diagnosis of myocardial necrosis. It is even more specific for myocardium than CKMB; its release is independent of perfusion; there is only slow extracellular elimination, intracellular degradation is unknown; in normal conditions it is not detectable in the plasma, but there is a very large intracellular pool so even minor myocardial damage can be detected.

Evaluation of marker proteins as non-invasive indices of thrombolysis
Myosin light chain has been studied as a marker of reperfusion in a cohort of 44 patients. All had clinical and electrocardiographic evidence of myocardial infarction. Thirty-six patients were assigned to intracoronary thrombolytic therapy. Recanalization was achieved in eight patients within 3.5 hours; these patients constituted the early reperfusion (ER) group. In another 18 patients, reperfusion was achieved after more than 3.5 hours; these constituted the late reperfusion (LR) group. In ten patients streptokinase infusion did not result in reperfusion. These 10 patients, plus the eight not treated due to late admission or other contraindications to thrombolytic therapy,

constituted the permanent occlusion (PO) group. Blood samples were obtained at intervals following the onset of pain. Early reperfusion induced less marker protein release; this may be regarded as infarct size limitation. However, the time course of myosin light chain release was not different between the three groups. Hence, structural myocardial proteins, such as myosin light chain, do not seem suitable for identification of patients with successful thrombolysis.

Median serum concentrations of CK show a tendency towards an early rise in patients with early reperfusion compared to those with later reperfusion; this is even more apparent when compared to those with permanent occlusion. Much the same is true for CKMB, with earlier reperfusion inducing an earlier rise of CKMB; this profile is not very different from that obtained with late reperfusion, whereas in patients with permanent occlusion CKMB is only released after some delay. Myoglobin gives the best distinction between patients with early and late reperfusion. The slowest rise of protein plasma concentration of myoglobin was again observed in patients with permanent occlusion.

For CK, CKMB and myoglobin, the time for peak concentration depends on the time reperfusion is established. The earlier reperfusion occurs, the earlier the peak plasma level is attained. The time to peak value of CK is about three to four times longer than the reperfusion time; that is, for a reperfusion time of five hours, the time to peak CK level is around 15-20 hours. The correlation coefficient is 0.65. With CKMB the interval between recanalization and reperfusion is likely to be shorter. With reperfusion at five hours, the time to peak plasma CKMB is about 10-15 hours; the correlation coefficient is 0.71. The best results are obtained with myoglobin. The time interval between recanalization and marker protein release is the shortest, with a correlation coefficient of 0.94.

Time to peak CK level offers good discrimination between reperfusion occurring within 12 hours and permanent occlusion (with a peak value after 24 hours and more). In the period 12-24 hours, however, reperfused and non-reperfused myocardial infarction cannot be discriminated on the basis of peak CK levels. Univariate analysis may be undertaken to determine the probability of correct classification of infarct reperfusion. Optimal discriminatory time limit for infarct reperfusion corresponds to a probability of 0.5. This corresponds to a time of 16 hours, with a probability of correct classification of 89%.

For myoglobin, the results are even better. The optimal discriminatory time limit, allowing a probability of 0.5, is about seven to eight hours. In these circumstances there is 93% probability of correct classification of reperfused and non-reperfused myocardium.

The predictive value of peak plasma levels of marker protein in discriminating between reperfused and non-reperfused myocardium can be enhanced by using two proteins. To take CK and myoglobin as examples, the combined use of time to peak concentration for both proteins discriminates extremely well between reperfused and non-reperfused myocardium, and is better than either protein alone for this purpose.

CAUSES OF EARLY MORTALITY: RUPTURE AND ARRHYTHMIA

D.G. JULIAN

Rupture has been a much neglected aspect of myocardial infarction. Physicians have, perhaps appropriately, taken a rather fatalistic attitude towards it, but have not realized how frequent an event rupture is and what might be done to prevent it.

Types of cardiac rupture

There is much misunderstanding of the pathology of rupture. Becker & Van Mantgem [1], in 1975, classified rupture into three different types. Type 1 was a slit-like tear that usually occurred within the first 24 hours after myocardial infarction in a ventricle which was often quite good and frequently had no previous infarction in it. Type 2 rupture involved erosion of infarcted myocardium, with a variable time of onset of symptoms. Type 3 rupture was associated with early aneurysm formation, but it could occur days or even weeks after the acute event. Type 1 rupture is much the most common.

Rates of cardiac rupture

Cardiac rupture may be responsible for one-quarter of all deaths in a coronary care unit [1]. Interest in rupture was stimulated by data from the ISIS-I trial of beta-blockade [2]. ISIS-I studied the effect of intravenous and oral beta-blockade on prognosis after acute myocardial infarction, and a rather unexpected finding emerged. At seven days, there was a significant reduction in mortality in the atenolol group compared to the control group; when a retrospective analysis was done, however, it appeared that this benefit was confined almost exclusively to the first day or two (that is, the day of symptom onset and the day afterwards). The apparent lack of benefit from day three to day seven was puzzling, as it did not seem to correspond with the original concept that the treatment would reduce infarct size and produce a late benefit as well as an early benefit. There also appears to have been a reduction in rupture in the similar MIAMI study [3].

In the light of this finding, it was felt that a review should be made of the records of those patients who had died in the first two days. These records were not available from all countries, so the study concentrated on the United Kingdom, Ireland and Scandinavia (Table 1). Quite a large number of these individuals died with electro-mechanical dissociation, that is, continuing electrical activity in the absence of mechanical function; 54 patients in the control group and 20 in the atenolol group died in that way. In virtually all of those patients who demonstrated electro-mechanical dissociation and on whom autopsies were subsequently performed, cardiac rupture was demonstrated — 17 in the control group, five in the atenolol group. In 37 control group patients and 15 atenolol group patients, autopsy was not performed but the clinical picture was one of electro-mechanical dissociation.

There were slight differences in the causes of death between the two groups, but when all deaths attributable to mechanical causes were pooled, the numbers involved

Footnote. The author wishes to express his gratitude to Professor Michael Davies, St George's Hospital, London, for advice on this presentation.

Table 1. Mode of death among patients receiving atenolol or control dying during days 0-1 of ISIS-I in UK, Ireland and Scandinavia only.

	Deaths during days 0-1	
Mode of death	Atenolol group	Control group
Cardiac deaths without mechanical failure		
Cardiac rupture confirmed by necrospy	5	17*
Electro-mechanical dissociation	15	37 †
1° ventricular fibrillation	5	13
Bradycardia/asystole	10	3
Cardiac deaths with mechanical failure		
Shock	34	24
Left ventricular failure	6	13
Non-cardiac deaths		
Respiratory arrest	3	0
Aortic dissection	1	5
Cerebrovascular accident	0	2
Deaths without review of clinical records	12	12
UK, Ireland, and Scandinavia only		
Total deaths in days 0-1	91	126*
No. randomised	6121	6101
Other countries		
Total deaths in days 0-1	30	45
No. randomised	1916	1889

*2p <0.01; † 2p > 0.01.

were found to be roughly similar for both groups. Somewhat more people in the atenolol group succumbed to shock; conversely, there were more instances of ventricular failure in the control group. The high frequency of shock in the atenolol group may be attributed to the reduction in blood pressure effected by this drug, giving rise to a clinical picture compatible with the definition of shock employed in the study. Overall then, the effect of treatment on ventricular function did not seem to be very great, and the early benefit accruing from beta-blocker treatment appeared to be due to prevention of early rupture, presumably Type 1.

Risk factors for cardiac rupture
Within this, admittedly limited, number of patients, how did those at particularly high risk for rupture fare? Rupture has been recognized as being a relatively common event in women as opposed to men, in the elderly as opposed to the younger patient, and in the hypertensive or normotensive subject as opposed to the hypotensive patient. Subsetting is a rather dubious practise, but it is of interest to look at the kind of figures that emerge from ISIS-I. There was a higher death rate in the hypertensive control group than among atenolol treated hypertensives (4.3% versus 2.9%). The differential was less marked in normotensives and, if anything, treatment had an adverse effect in

patients with hypotension. These data do, however, appear to confirm hypertension as a risk factor for cardiac rupture, and they indicate that atenolol is a means of preventing death from this mechanism.

Rupture is also a function of age and in the older age group the benefit of atenolol is more apparent than in the younger age group. Likewise, the benefit of treatment is apparently greater in females than in males. All this information tends to support the view that the mechanism of prevention of death by atenolol, or at least the major mechanism, relates to the prevention of rupture.

Influence of thrombolytic therapy

It is also interesting to consider thrombolytic therapy and its effect on rupture. In the ISIS-II trial there was very little difference in rates of rupture between the treated and control groups; the same is true of GISSI-I. In GISSI-I there was some evidence of an increase in rupture on the first day in the treated group, followed by a subsequent decrease, so that the overall amount of rupture was roughly the same.

The ISIS-II data has yet to be fully analysed but preliminary figures are available. On the first day, around 30 patients on streptokinase died from cardiac rupture compared to 18 in the placebo group. Following these groups through to day 35, there was little difference between them, suggesting, as in GISSI-I, that streptokinase may increase the rate of rupture on the first day but decrease it on subsequent days. There was little difference in rates of rupture between the placebo and aspirin groups on day 1, with 20 deaths in the placebo group and 25 in the aspirin group. At the end of 35 days, however, there was a reduced incidence of rupture in patients on aspirin, although this was not a significant reduction. With combined streptokinase and aspirin there was a more marked suggestion of an increase of rupture on the first day — five in the control group, 14 in the streptokinase plus aspirin group. Over time, this trend reversed so that there were more ruptures in the placebo group than in the streptokinase and aspirin group.

These results need more detailed analysis, and although the differences are not statistically significant, the data does tend to support the suggestion that streptokinase or other thrombolytic agents will increase rupture on the first day and decrease it subsequently, thus perhaps increasing the incidence of Type 1 rupture and decreasing the incidence of Type 3 rupture.

Pooling the ISIS-I and ISIS-II data, it could be argued that there is a very strong case for combining beta-blockade and streptokinase for the purpose of preventing rupture on the first day. At present this is entirely speculative, but the proposal does serve to focus attention on rupture, a major cause of death.

References

[1] Becker AE, van Mantgem J-P.
     Cardiac tamponade.
     Eur J Cardiol 1975; **3/4**: 359–71.

[2] ISIS-I Collaborative Group.
     Mechanisms for the early mortality
     reduction produced by beta-blockade started
     early in acute myocardial infarction: ISIS-I.
     Lancet 1988; **i**: 921–3.

[3] The MIAMI Trial Research Group.
     Development of myocardial infarction.
     Am J Cardiol 1985; **56**: 239–69.

4. ADJUVANT STRATEGIES: MEDICAL INTERVENTIONS

THE ROLE OF BETA-BLOCKERS, CALCIUM ANTAGONISTS AND NITRATES IN ACUTE MYOCARDIAL INFARCTION

C. COWAN

Thrombolysis represents one mechanism of infarct size limitation, acting on the supply side of the supply:demand equation. Beta-blockers, calcium antagonists and nitrates act primarily on the demand side, with the similar aim of infarct size limitation. Studies on these agents predate studies on thrombolytic therapy — they virtually belong to an earlier decade — and it is appropriate to review briefly our existing knowledge of the role of beta-blockers, calcium antagonists and nitrates in acute myocardial infarction before discussing to what extent this data can be extrapolated into the thrombolytic era.

Studies on beta-blockers, calcium antagonists and nitrates
Fig. 1 presents a meta-analysis of data from studies on acute beta-blockade, calcium antagonists and nitrates. An odds ratio <1 represents a benefit of treatment; an odds

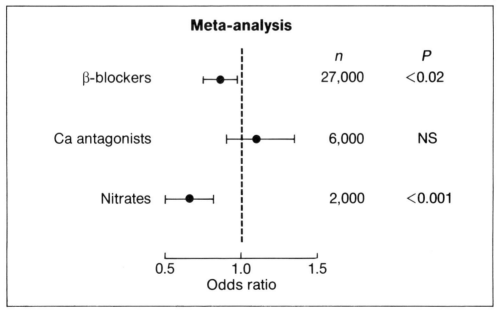

Fig. 1.   Meta-analysis of randomised studies of beta-blockers, calcium antagonists and nitrates in acute infarction. An odds ratio <1 indicates a lower mortality in the active treatment group, and an odds ratio >1 indicates a higher mortality in the active treatment group. 95% Confidence limits are shown. n indicates the total number of patients randomised to active treatment or control. For further information see references 1, 2, and 3.

ratio >1 represents an adverse effect. This data arises *solely* from studies dealing with intervention in acute myocardial infarction, and does not include any evaluation of these agents in long-term prophylaxis post-myocardial infarction. In the case of beta-blockers, some 27,000 patients have been randomized. The mean benefit is a 13% reduction in mortality, which is just significant [1]. Some 6000 patients have been randomized to calcium antagonists. Pooling shows a small adverse effect of treatment, which is not statistically significant [2]. The result for nitrates is perhaps the most surprising. Pooling of data yields a mortality reduction of around 35%; this is highly significant [3]. Hence, meta-analysis suggests that nitrates have a considerably greater benefit than either beta-blockers or calcium antagonists. However, this conclusion should be treated with great caution. The number of patients who have been randomised in studies of intravenous nitrates is relatively small — a mere 2000. If there have been any studies with less favourable results which have gone unreported, the overall results might look much less favourable.

Not everyone may be happy with the principles of meta-analysis, so a brief consideration of the results of a few individual investigations is appropriate.

1.   Fig. 2 shows data drawn from the ISIS-I study [4]. This study showed a reduction in mortality of 15% in atenolol-treated patients over controls. Most of the reduction in mortality was achieved over the first two days of the study.

2.   In the TRENT study [5] there was no reduction in mortality of patients treated with nifedipine (Fig. 3).

3.   Results from the largest of the studies of intravenous glyceryl trinitrate [6] are shown in Fig. 4. The study is still a small one, randomizing a mere 300 patients to treatment. A marked reduction in mortality was seen amongst treated patients. However, it is worth noting that not only were small total numbers involved in this study, but mortality in the control group was very high — 30% at one year.

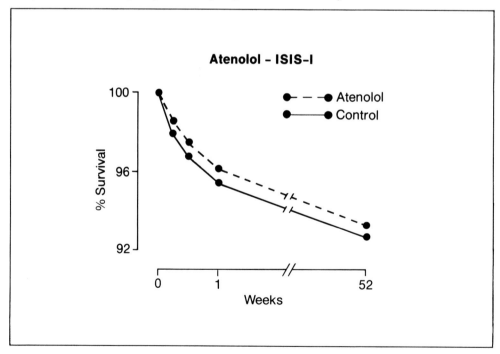

Fig. 2.   Effects of beta-blockade on mortality in acute myocardial infarction. (After ISIS-I Study Group. *Lancet* 1986; **ii:** 57–65. [4])

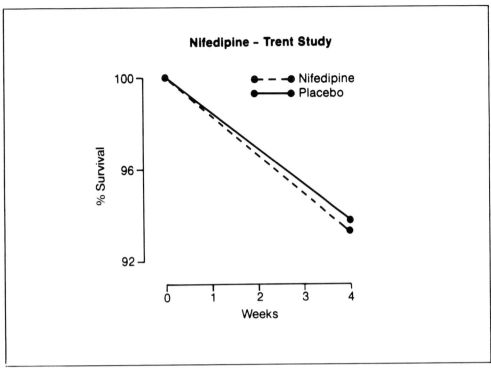

Fig. 3. Lack of effect of calcium antagonists on mortality in acute myocardial infarction. (After Wilcox RG, Hampton JR, Banks DC, *et al. Br Med J* 1986; **293:** 1204–8. [5])

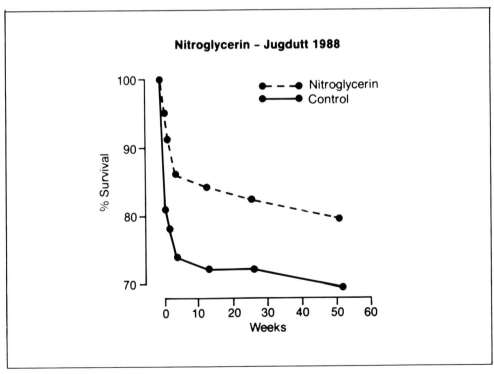

Fig. 4. Effects of nitrates on mortality in acute myocardial infarction. (After Jugdutt BI, Warnica JW. *Circulation* 1988; **78:** 906–19. [6])

Combination therapy in acute myocardial infarction

Do any of these agents yield an additive benefit when combined with thrombolytic agents? The extent of mortality reduction with single factor interventions is shown in Fig. 5. To what extent can these single factor mortality reductions be summated? Certainly in the case of aspirin and streptokinase the effects are additive — from ISIS-II data, these agents produce a combined mortality reduction of 42%. However, it is not known if beta-blockers will prevent a further 15% of deaths, as atenolol did in ISIS-I. This would bring the cumulative mortality reduction to 51%. If a nitrate were then to be added, would it bring the cumulative mortality reduction to 68%? Finally, would the further addition of heparin bring the cumulative mortality reduction to 73%?

Many clinicians would be deeply sceptical of the possibility of reducing mortality in acute myocardial infarction by nearly three-quarters. Nevertheless, there are good reasons to believe that at least partial additive effects of therapy may exist.

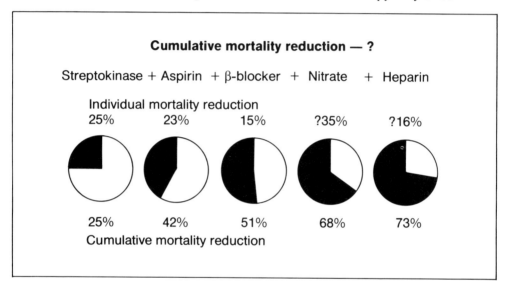

Fig. 5. Is the mortality reduction with different interventions additive? The individual mortality reductions which have been demonstrated for different interventions, or inferred from meta-analysis, are shown in the upper row of figures. The pie graphs indicate the cumulative mortality reduction (shaded area), if we assume that these interventions are additive. Thus, if the effects of aspirin and streptokinase are additive, aspirin would prevent 23% of the 75% of deaths still occurring after streptokinase, giving a cumulative mortality reduction of 42%. This cumulative benefit of aspirin and streptokinase was confirmed in the ISIS-II study. The cumulative benefits of beta-blockade, nitrates and heparin are, by contrast, speculative.

Beta-blockers

Considering beta-blockers first, a number of animal studies have suggested that beta-blocker therapy to limit infarct size may be more successful when accompanying reperfusion than when given with a maintained occlusion. Fig. 6 illustrates one such study [7], in which infarct size was determined after occlusion of a lateral circumflex coronary artery in dogs. With maintained occlusion,propranolol failed to reduce infarct size. However, with reperfusion at one hour, propranolol substantially reduced infarct size. It may be anticipated, therefore, that beta-blockers would be more effective when accompanying thrombolytic therapy.

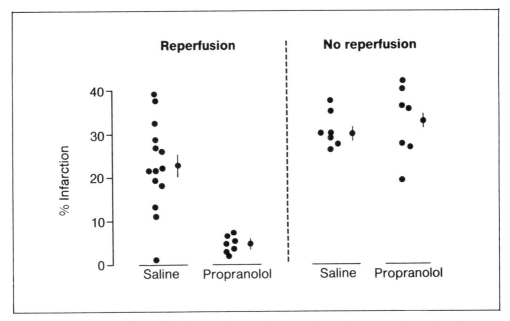

Fig. 6. Interaction of beta-blockade and reperfusion. Infarct size was estimated as the percentage of the left ventricle infarcted following coronary ligation in dogs. With maintained occlusion, propranolol reduced infarct size. With reperfusion (through a critical stenosis) after ligation for 60 minutes, propranolol reduced infarct size. (Reproduced with permission from Reynolds RD, Burmeister WD, Gorczynski RJ, Dickerson DD, Mathews MP, Lee RJ. *Cardiovasc Res* 1981; **15**: 411–20. [7])

Some insight may be gained into whether effects are likely to be additive by considering the mechanism through which beta-blockers reduce mortality. Retrospective analysis was conducted for causes of death in about 200 patients dying in the first two days of the ISIS-I study (the period during which most of the benefit of atenolol treatment was seen) [8]. The reduced mortality rate in the treatment group was almost entirely due to a decreased incidence of left ventricular rupture (or presumed rupture, as evidenced by electro-mechanical dissociation). This reduction in left ventricular rupture might well be additive to the benefits of thrombolytic agents. ISIS-II data shows that mortality in the aspirin/streptokinase treated patients was *not* reduced in the first two days of treatment [9]. Therefore, it may reasonably be expected that the beta-blocker effect on left ventricular rupture would be additive during this interval.

The issue of the possible benefits of the combination of beta-blockade with thrombolysis was addressed in the TIMI-II study [10]. While the main objective of this investigation was to assess various strategies of angioplasty, a subsidiary objective was to assess the impact of beta-blockade, in combination with thrombolytic therapy, on mortality.

Of the 3000 patients receiving t-PA, 1390 were randomized to strategies of immediate or deferred beta-blockade. There was no difference in ejection fraction between the two groups at 42 days. There was no effect on mortality, although it is worth emphasizing that this study was too small to expect to pick up any mortality benefit. There were borderline benefits in recurrence of ischaemia and reinfarction at six days, but by 42 days these benefits were no longer statistically significant.

The authors placed some emphasis on subgroup analysis. They found that patients treated within two hours of onset of symptoms showed a statistically significant reduction in a pooled end-point of death or reinfarction, whereas no benefit was evident with treatment initiated after two hours. Subgroup analysis of such small numbers is only useful as a pointer for further studies, or to look for similar benefits in equivalent subgroups in other studies. This early treatment subgroup is of interest because a similar marked benefit was observed in patients treated within two hours in ISIS-I [4]. It may well be that very early beta-blockade is of particular benefit and that this benefit is additive to thrombolytic therapy.

The second TIMI subgroup considered was a grouping into low-risk and non-low-risk patients. In brief, patients in the low-risk category were young, had no history of previous myocardial infarction and had an uncomplicated inferior infarct. This low-risk cohort showed considerable benefits when treated with beta-blockers, whereas there was a slight and non-significant rise in mortality in the non-low-risk subgroup. The significance of these results is more controversial. They do not seem consistent with those in other studies — for example, in the MIAMI study it was the high-risk subgroup which particularly benefitted from beta-blocker therapy [11].

Overall, the conclusion from TIMI-II has to be that this is not the definitive study. To further assess the possible additive benefits of thrombolysis and beta-blockade, much larger studies will be necessary. A note of caution is necessary, however. Despite the proven benefits of beta-blockade in acute myocardial infarction, physician acceptance of this treatment has been variable. In the GISSI-II study, 46% of patients were treated with intravenous beta-blockade. This is in marked contrast to clinical practice in Great Britain which has remained essentially unchanged, despite the benefits of intravenous beta-blockers demonstrated in ISIS-I. So, even if it is shown that beta-blockers have an additive effect, would this demonstration influence clinical practice? Certainly in Great Britain, a change in the attitude of physicians would also be necessary.

Calcium antagonists

As discussed earlier, the existing studies on the use of calcium antagonists in acute infarction have not suggested any mortality benefit. These studies predate the thrombolytic era and the question remains open whether calcium antagonists might still be of benefit in combination with thrombolytics.

Nitrates

Some of the possible mechanisms of action of nitrates are obvious — reduction in preload, reduction in afterload, stenosis dilatation. Early treatment with intravenous nitrates has also been shown to prevent late infarct expansion [6]. There is, in addition, the controversial possibility that nitrates may have an anti-platelet effect. In the last few years, evidence has been accumulating that the actions of nitrates are mediated through the genesis of nitric oxide. There is also increasing evidence that nitric oxide is a naturally occurring vasodilator and that the agent for many years termed endothelium-derived relaxant factor (EDRF) is, in fact, nitric oxide [12]. EDRF, in addition to its relaxant effect on vascular smooth muscle, is known to have anti-platelet effects (Fig. 7). Several reports have suggested that therapeutically administered nitrates may share this anti-platelet action, although this is controversial. If such an effect exists it would be of importance, because its pathway of action is cGMP dependent and therefore differs from the effects of aspirin, which are prostacyclin-mediated and cAMP dependent. Hence it is possible, although speculative, that nitrates may have an anti-platelet effect which would be additive to that of aspirin.

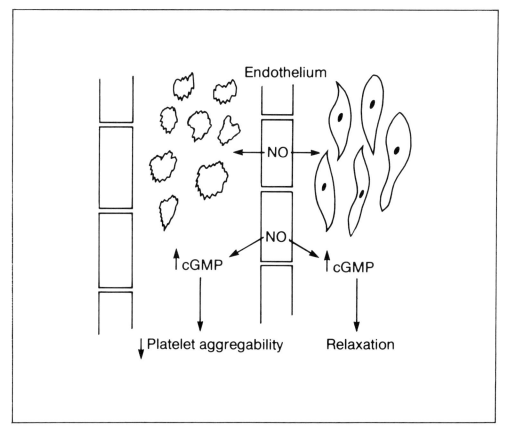

Fig. 7. Endothelium derived relaxing factor. Nitric oxide (NO) derived from the endothelium has both an intravascular platelet inhibitory effect and an extravascular smooth muscle relaxant action. Nitric oxide released intracellularly from therapeutically administered organic nitrates shares the action on smooth muscle, but effects on platelet aggregability are controversial.

Less speculative is the role of nitrates in stenosis dilatation. Nitrates can also influence the supply side of the supply:demand equation. Professor Maseri (see page 29) has emphasized that reperfusion is not an all-or-none event, but a 'stuttering' one. Fig. 8 presents an example of this from our own work. A patient was found to have reperfused on coronary angiography 60 minutes after the administration of t-PA. However, by 90 min the coronary artery had reoccluded. At this stage intracoronary isosorbide dinitrate was given and reperfusion was restored. This suggests there is synergism between thrombolytics and nitrates in achieving early reperfusion, indicating possible additive benefits.

Conclusion

There are reasons to believe that both beta-blockers and nitrates may bestow additive benefits when used to complement reperfusion strategies. Physician acceptance of early intravenous beta-blockade has been variable. Nitrates, by contrast, are already commonly used in acute infarction. Further studies are needed to determine whether their use, in combination with thrombolytic therapy, should be adopted as standard practice.

Post t-PA   60 min

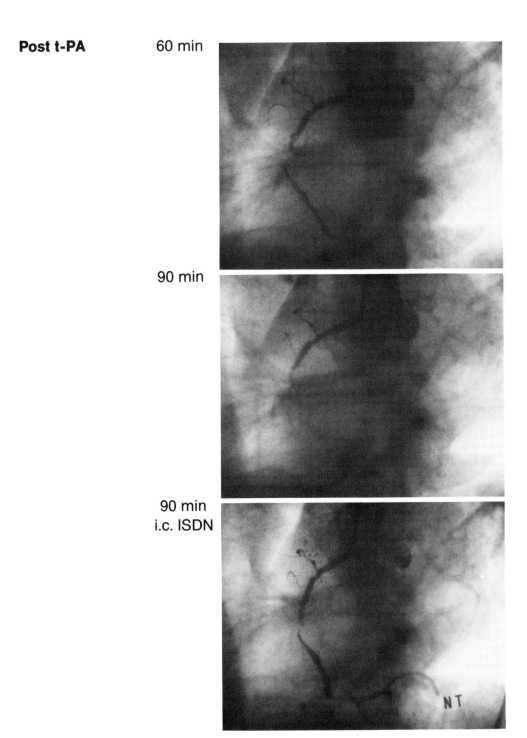

90 min

90 min
i.c. ISDN

Fig. 8. Synergism between nitrates and thrombolytics. Right coronary injections are shown at varying time intervals after the systemic administration of t-PA. At 60 minutes, reperfusion has occurred. At 90 minutes, the artery has reoccluded. Following the i.c. administration of isosorbide dinitrate, perfusion is restored.

References

[1] Yusuf S, Peto R, Lewis J, Collins R, Sleight P.
Beta blockade during and after myocardial infarction: an overview of the randomized trials.
Progr Cardiovasc Dis 1985; **27**: 335–71.

[2] Yusuf S, Furberg CD.
Effects of calcium channel blockers on survival after myocardial infarction.
Cardiovasc Drugs Ther 1987; **1**: 343–4.

[3] Yusuf S, Collins R, MacMahon S, Peto R.
Effect of intravenous nitrates on mortality in acute myocardial infarction: an overview of the randomised trials.
Lancet 1988; **i**: 1088–92.

[4] ISIS-I Study Group.
Randomised trial of intravenous atenolol among 16027 cases of suspected acute myocardial infarction: ISIS-I.
Lancet 1986; **ii**: 57–65.

[5] Wilcox RG, Hampton JR, Banks DC, *et al.*
Trial of early nifedipine in acute myocardial infarction: the Trent study.
Br Med J 1986; **293**: 1204–8.

[6] Jugdutt BI, Warnica JW.
Intravenous nitroglycerin therapy to limit myocardial infarct size, expansion and complications. Effect of timing, dosage and infarct location.
Circulation 1988; **78**: 906–19.

[7] Reynolds RD, Burmeister WD, Gorczynski RJ, Dickerson DD, Mathews MP, Lee RJ.
Effects of propranolol on myocardial infarct size with and without coronary artery reperfusion in the dog.
Cardiovasc Res 1981; **15**: 411–20.

[8] ISIS-I Study Group.
Mechanisms for the early mortality reduction produced by beta-blockade started early in acute myocardial infarction: ISIS-I.
Lancet 1988; **i**: 921–3.

[9] ISIS-II Study Group.
Randomised trial of intravenous streptokinase, oral aspirin, both, or neither among 17187 cases of suspected acute myocardial infarction: ISIS-II.
Lancet 1988; **ii**: 349–60.

[10] TIMI Study Group.
Comparison of invasive and conservative strategies after treatment with intravenous tissue plasminogen activator in acute myocardial infarction. Results of the thrombolysis in myocardial infarction (TIMI) phase II trial.
N Engl J Med 1989; **320;** 618–27.

[11] MIAMI Trial Research Group.
Metoprolol in acute myocardial infarction (MIAMI). A randomized placebo controlled international trial.
Eur Heart J 1985; **6**: 199–226.

[12] Griffith TM, Lewis MJ, Newby AC, Henderson AH.
Endothelium-derived relaxing factor.
J Am Coll Cardiol 1988; **12**: 797–806.

[13] Hackett D, Davies G, Chierchia S, Maseri A.
Intermittent coronary occlusion in acute myocardial infarction. Value of combined thrombolytic and vasodilator therapy.
N Engl J Med 1987; **317**: 1055–9.

ASPIRIN AND OTHER ANTI-PLATELET AGENTS IN ACUTE MYOCARDIAL INFARCTION

P. SLEIGHT

Fresh thrombus formation is a very dynamic affair; even while thrombus is being lysed, it is reclotting again. It is reasonable to speculate that aspirin may be helpful in arresting this process. The conclusions from an overview of the antiplatelet trials in secondary prevention (post-myocardial infarction, post-transient ischaemic attacks) and in unstable angina were so striking that it seemed worthwhile trying aspirin in the treatment of acute myocardial infarction in ISIS-II.

The ISIS-II study
Since thrombus formation is a dynamic process from onset, it seemed appropriate for patients to chew the first tablet as there is some buccal absorption from chewed aspirin; aspirin might not be so well absorbed from the stomach in patients who have been given morphine and opiates. The dose was empirically chosen at 160 mg of enteric coated aspirin.

Mortality rates
The results are now well known but at the time of the trial it was a surprise to find that aspirin had such a powerful effect — nearly as good as thrombolytic therapy alone. Moreover, the effect of aspirin plus streptokinase was additive. Fig. 1 shows the ISIS-II data for five-week mortality: aspirin reduced the odds of dying by 23% when com-

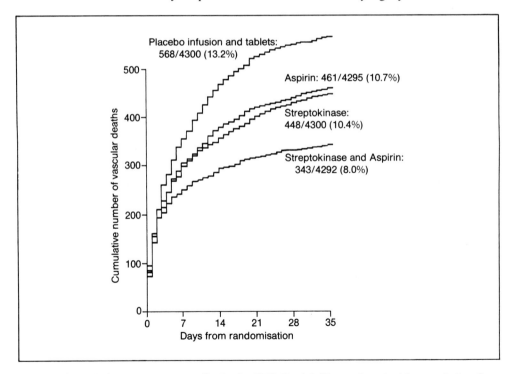

Fig. 1. Cumulative vascular mortality in the ISIS-II trial. (Reproduced with permission from ISIS-II Collaborative Group, *Lancet* 1988; **ii:** 349–60.)

pared to placebo. As Fig. 2 shows, aspirin was active in all groups of patients categorized according to the location of infarct. This is quite an important point since one criticism of ISIS-II results has been that the benefits of aspirin therapy were due to its influence on unstable angina. Fig. 2 makes it clear that aspirin worked equally well in all classes of patients. Unlike the response to thrombolysis, no time-dependent gradient was observed for aspirin. There was no evidence that aspirin was harmful in the older patients; indeed, if anything, it appeared to confer greater benefit in these patients though this did not attain statistical significance.

	Aspirin	Placebo tablets	Odds ratio & 95% CI	
			Aspirin better	Placebo better
Entry ECG				
BBB	74/ 407 (18.2%)	111/ 420 (26.4%)		
Inf ST elev	147/2081 (7.1%)	188/2107 (8.9%)		
Ant ST elev	236/1847 (12.8%)	300/1815 (16.5%)		
I & A ST elev	19/ 150 (12.7%)	21/ 166 (12.7%)		
ST depression	103/ 578 (17.8%)	109/ 559 (19.5%)		
Other abn.	89/1983 (4.5%)	107/1974 (5.4%)		
'Normal' ECG	5/ 156 (3.2%)	4/ 159 (2.5%)		
All patients	804/8587 (9.4%)	1016/8600 (11.8%)		23% SD4 odds reduction

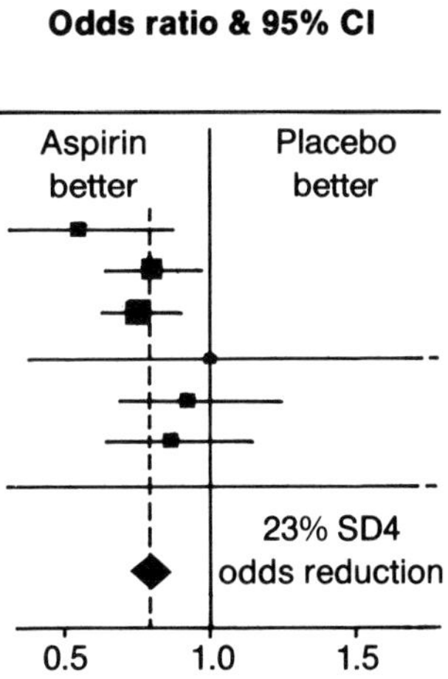

0.5 1.0 1.5

Fig. 2. Effects of aspirin on five-week vascular mortality — subdivided by entry ECG — in ISIS-II. (Redrawn with permission from ISIS-II Collaborative Group, *Lancet* 1988; **ii:** 349–60.)

Reinfarction rates

In the double placebo cohort of ISIS-II, there was a 3% incidence of clinically-diagnosed reinfarction during the period of hospital in-patient stay. Given the relatively crude criteria applied, this is probably an underestimate of the incidence of reinfarction and is certainly a gross underestimate of the incidence of reocclusion. As might have been expected on the basis of other studies, reinfarction rates during the in-patient stay were increased in patients receiving streptokinase alone (from 3% to 4%). With the combined streptokinase and aspirin regimen, however, the reinfarction rate was reduced to only 2%, similar to that seen in the aspirin only group (Table 1). Thus, the addition of aspirin appears to eliminate the excess of reinfarction caused by thrombolytic therapy. It should be noted though, that this still leaves at least a 2%

Table 1. Reinfarction rates with aspirin and streptokinase in ISIS-II.

	Active SK	Placebo infusion
Active aspirin	77 (2%)	79 (2%)
Placebo tablets	161 (4%)	123 (3%)

incidence of infarction that may be attributed to mechanisms not affected by aspirin treatment. Possibly nitrates or some of the newer anti-platelet agents may have a contribution to make here.

Side-effects

Aspirin was very safe. There was no excess of major bleeds in the group that received aspirin and streptokinase compared to streptokinase alone, and there was just a 1% excess of minor bleeds and bruising in those given combined therapy. In addition, there was no aggravation of other side-effects.

So, for in-hospital events, aspirin was associated with no increase in serious bleeding, a 40% reduction in stroke, and a 49% (from 3.3% to 1.8%) reduction in reinfarction. Aspirin was also remarkably well tolerated. Discontinuation of therapy while in hospital amounted to 7% of patients in both groups, so there is no evidence that more patients in the active aspirin groups were discontinuing aspirin because of indigestion or other side-effects. The effect of aspirin, like the effect of streptokinase, was sustained for up to two years (median time 15 months).

The overall 'balance sheet' for aspirin is that among 100 patients treated acutely and then followed for two to three years, there are four fewer deaths and four fewer major events (such as stroke or non-fatal infarction) than among patients not receiving aspirin.

Recent therapeutic trends

Between 1987 and 1989 there has been a very great increase in the proportion of physicians using both anti-platelet and fibrinolytic therapies (Collins R & Julian DJ, personal communication). The results of really large trials such as ISIS-II and GISSI do clearly influence doctors' attitudes — clinical practice in the UK has probably altered faster than ever before.

This is not to say that the influence of trials has been entirely beneficent. One of the greatest perils is that of incorrect interpretation of results from sub-group analysis. Taking inferior myocardial infarction as an example, it could be said that patients have died as a result of such analyses. Doctors believed that the finding of no significant benefit in a trial meant that treatment of inferior infarction conferred no benefit at all, with the result that many people with such infarcts were not treated. Subsequent analysis of pooled data has dispelled this belief.

What about anticoagulants? In the mid-1980s, differences in national practise between the USA and UK made it impractical to organize a properly randomized study of the effect of heparin on aspirin-treated patients within ISIS-II, but inspection of the data available from that trial indicates a trend towards improved odds in patients given streptokinase and aspirin plus anticoagulant therapy with intravenous heparin. ISIS-III and GISSI-II will look into this more systematically, using high dose subcutaneous calcium heparin administered twice-daily. In the recently published McMaster trial, this regime significantly reduced the incidence of left ventricular thrombosis in acute myocardial infarction when compared with the conventional 'low dose' of 5000 U of subcutaneous heparin twice-daily.

There have been few direct, randomized comparisons of aspirin dose. From an overview of secondary prevention trials, it appears that large doses of aspirin are no better than one aspirin per day. Certainly, the UK TIA study chaired by Prof. Charles

Warlow reported a tripling of minor and serious side-effects when high dose (1200 mg) aspirin was used, and there appeared to be no offsetting therapeutic gain from the high dose compared to low dose (300 mg).

Trials of aspirin plus dipyridamole versus aspirin alone suggest no additional benefit of the combined therapies, but patient numbers have been limited and more data will be needed to substantiate these findings. To judge from experience in ISIS-II, there are no patients in whom aspirin is not effective and it should be used in all patients unless there are strong contraindications. Optimal dosage appears to lie between 160 mg and 325 mg. Information on lower doses, for example 60-100 mg aspirin/day, suggest benefit but there is not enough evidence to be dogmatic about whether these much lower doses are as effective as 160-325 mg aspirin/day.

EFFECTIVENESS OF ANTICOAGULANT THERAPY IN REDUCING MORBIDITY AND MORTALITY IN ACUTE MYOCARDIAL INFARCTION

J. HIRSH

Few subjects have engendered as much controversy as the use of anticoagulants in acute myocardial infarction. Anticoagulant therapy was used routinely in the treatment of acute myocardial infarction in the 1950s and 1960s. Its popularity began to wane in the early 1970s after publication of several studies evaluating anticoagulant therapy in the treatment of acute myocardial infarction [1-13]. Review of the evidence suggests that neither the initial enthusiastic support for anticoagulants nor their subsequent rejection was justified by the published reports.

Clinical trials have evaluated anticoagulants for the early long-term treatment of acute myocardial infarction, for the treatment of unstable angina, and as an adjunct to thrombolytic therapy in the treatment of acute myocardial infarction. In this presentation, I will concentrate on the randomized trials that enrolled sufficient patient numbers to be able to demonstrate clinically important differences in mortality, reinfarction, systemic embolism or pulmonary embolism.

Rationale for the short-term use of anticoagulants
The early use of anticoagulants in patients with acute myocardial infarction has the potential to:

1. Prevent extension or recurrence of coronary artery thrombosis and to reduce infarct size and prevent reinfarction;
2. Prevent mural thrombosis and its complication, systemic embolism;
3. Prevent the development of venous thrombosis and pulmonary embolism.

It is clear from the results of recent studies using coronary angiography that 80%-90% of patients with acute myocardial infarction have an occlusive thrombus at presentation and, therefore, that the thrombus is already present before anticoagulant therapy can be commenced [14]. Even if anticoagulants can prevent the extension of coronary artery thrombosis, it is unlikely that they will modify infarct size, which is the major determinant of early mortality in patients who are admitted to hospital with acute myocardial infarction. It is possible, however, that anticoagulants can reduce the frequency of reinfarction by reducing the frequency of rethrombosis in coronary arteries that have recanalized spontaneously. Anticoagulants may be more effective in reducing the frequency of systemic embolism and pulmonary embolism, but these two complications of myocardial infarction are uncommon causes of serious morbidity or mortality and, therefore, their reduction will have only a relatively minor influence on mortality in acute myocardial infarction.

Since 1948, there have been over 30 reports on the use of anticoagulants in acute myocardial infarction [15]. Three of the studies were randomized trials which were relatively large [1-3], but none were of sufficient size to have an 80% chance of demonstrating a true reduction of 20%. Since subsequent experience with anticoagulants indicates that the expected improvement in mortality or reinfarction attributable to anticoagulants is likely to be in the range of 20%, all three studies lacked the statistical power necessary to demonstrate a realistic and clinically important effect. Details of the three large randomized trials are summarized below.

Medical Research Council [1]
This study was a single-blind, controlled trial in which 1427 patients of either sex with acute myocardial infarction were randomized on admission into an anticoagulant or comparison group and followed for a 28-day period. Patients assigned to the anticoagulant group received intravenous heparin in an initial 15,000 unit bolus followed by 10,000 units every six hours for up to five doses. Phenindione therapy was commenced at the same time and both anticoagulants were administered for 36 hours. Phenindione was adjusted to maintain the thrombotest level between 20% and 10% (INR = 1.6-2.1). The comparison group received no heparin but was given a homeopathic dose (1 mg) of phenindione. The total case fatality rates (at 28 days) were 18% in the comparative group and 16.2% in the anticoagulant group. Reinfarction (at 28 days) occurred in 13% of patients in the comparative group and 9.7% of patients in the high-dose anticoagulant group. Thus, the combined end-points of mortality and reinfarction occurred in 31% of patients in the comparative group and in 25.9% of patients in the high-dose anticoagulant group (a 16% reduction, which was not statistically significant). Patients receiving anticoagulants had a statistically significant lower incidence of clinically diagnosed pulmonary embolism (5.6% to 2.2%) and a significant reduction in stroke (2.5% to 1.1%). Haemorrhage was significantly more frequent in the anticoagulant group (5.1%) than in the comparative group (1.3%), but none of these haemorrhagic events was fatal.

Bronx Municipal Hospital Center Trial [2]
In this single-blind study, 1136 patients of both sexes with acute myocardial infarction were randomized to either an anticoagulant or placebo group within 24 hours of hospital admission. Patients in the anticoagulant group received 200 mg of phenindione and 5000 units of heparin intravenously. Heparin, 10,000 units subcutaneously, was then given every eight hours to a maximum of five doses and the dose of phenindione was adjusted to keep the prothrombin time between 2 and 2.5 times control (human brain thromboplastin) (INR = 2.0-2.5). The control group received an identical placebo. The case fatality rate was 21.2% in the control group and 14.9% in the group

receiving anticoagulants, a statistically significant difference ($P < 0.05$). On subgroup analysis, the effectiveness of anticoagulants appeared to be restricted to women. Reinfarction occurred in 13% of the control group and 11.8% of the treated group (not significant, NS). Pulmonary embolism (diagnosed clinically) occurred in 6.1% of patients in the control group and in 3.8% of those treated with anticoagulants (NS). Stroke occurred in 2.3% of control patients and 1.7% of those treated with anticoagulants (NS). There was a significantly higher frequency of haemorrhage in the anticoagulant group than in the control group, but none of these haemorrhagic complications was fatal.

Veterans Administration Cooperative Study [3]

In this trial, 999 men with acute myocardial infarction admitted to the Veterans Administration Hospitals throughout the United States were randomly allocated to treatment or placebo groups. Patients were entered within 72 hours of the onset of symptoms. The anticoagulant-treated group received heparin, 10,000 units subcutaneously, with further dosage adjustments according to the clotting time. Warfarin therapy was commenced at the same time and heparin was discontinued when the prothrombin time (human brain thromboplastin) was 25 seconds or greater (INR $>$ 2). Warfarin therapy was continued for 28 days. The control patients received identical placebo. The in-hospital mortality rates were 11.2% in the control group and 9.6% in the anticoagulant treatment group (NS). Reinfarction occurred in 4% of patients in the control group and 2% of patients in the anticoagulant-treated group (NS). Pulmonary embolism occurred in 2.6% of patients in the control group and in 0.2% of the group treated with anticoagulants ($P < 0.05$). Stroke was reported in 3.2% of patients in the control group and in 0.8% of the group receiving anticoagulants ($P < 0.05$).

Chalmers and associates [15], reanalysed the results of adequately designed, randomized studies of acute myocardial infarction and concluded that when the data were pooled there was an overall reduction in mortality of 21%.

Summary of effects of short-term anticoagulants on morbidity and mortality in acute myocardial infarction

Mortality

The results of the pooled analysis plus the trends in mortality rates in two of the three large studies and the significant reductions in mortality in the third, suggest that anticoagulants may produce a modest reduction of 20% (similar to the effect of aspirin) in early mortality in patients with acute myocardial infarction.

Most in-hospital deaths in patients admitted with acute myocardial infarction are caused by extensive myocardial damage or acute dysrhythmias. A relatively small proportion (approximately 10% of all deaths) are caused by systemic embolism (usually stroke) and an even smaller proportion are caused by pulmonary embolism. Therefore, it is not surprising that, in general, clinical trials have reported only a modest reduction in mortality attributable to anticoagulant therapy.

Systemic embolism

Systemic emboli arise from mural thrombi which form in the left ventricle at sites of hypokinesis or akinesis. Turpie et al. [16], showed that subcutaneous heparin in doses of 12,500 units 12-hourly was more effective than low dose heparin (in doses of 5,000 units 12-hourly) in preventing mural thrombosis as demonstrated by two-dimensional echocardiography in patients with acute myocardial infarction. The incidence of mural thrombosis was 31.8% in the low dose heparin group and 10.5% in the high dose group.

In the three large randomized studies [1-3], there was a statistically significant reduction in stroke in two (Table 1) and a non-significant trend in the third. The relative risk reduction for stroke in the anticoagulant treated group in these studies was 55% for the Medical Research Council Study ($P < 0.01$), 24% for the Bronx Municipal Hospital Centre Study (NS) and 75% for the Cooperative Veterans Administration Trial ($P < 0.001$). The results of these three large trials are supported by findings in smaller studies [8-22] and by the results of autopsy studies [20,21] (Tables 2 and 3), as well as by more recent reports.

Table 1.   Incidence of stroke in acute myocardial infarction.

Study	Regimen (no. of patients)	Stroke	Relative risk reduction (95% confidence limit)	P-value
VA Coop	Control (499)	0.032	75%	<0.005
	vs			
	coumarin (500)	0.008	(21% to 100%)	
MRC	Control (715)	0.025	55%	0.037
	vs			
	phenindione (712)	0.011	(0.5% to 100%)	

Table 2.   Thromboembolic complications of acute myocardial infarction.[+]

Thromboembolic complications	Heparin* (n = 105)	Placebo (n = 107)
Venous thromboembolism	7 (6.6%)	16 (14%)
Systemic embolism	3 (2.9%)	9 (8.4%)
Mural thrombosis (autopsy)	5	14

+ Steffensen, 1969
* Heparin 10,000 units b.i.d. subcutaneously

Table 3.   Thromboembolic complications at autopsy.*

Autopsy findings	Anticoagulant (371 patients, 85 dead, 84 autopsies)		No anticoagulant (427 patients, 109 dead, 92 autopsies)		P-value
Pulmonary embolism	4	5%	26	28%	0.01
Mural thrombosis	20	24%	53	58%	0.01

* Hilden et al. (1961). Prospective cohort study (level III)

The risk of stroke is between 1% and 3% for all infarctions and between 2% and 6% for patients with anterior myocardial infarction [23-28].

Patients at high risk of systemic embolism are those with anterior infarction, especially in the presence of wall motion abnormalities [23,26,29]. In this group of patients, the prevalence of left ventricular thrombosis is approximately 30%-40% [26,29,30]. Other risk factors are large infarct size, presence of a dilated and poorly functioning left ventricle, atrial fibrillation, cardiac failure and acute ventricular aneurysm. Patients with inferior infarcts are at low risk for systemic embolism. Most systemic thromboembolic events occur within the first three months of acute infarction.

The results of several small studies suggest an association between systemic embolism and mural thrombosis detected by two-dimensional echocardiography [23].

The intensity of anticoagulant therapy required to prevent arterial embolism is uncertain, but most studies used full doses of heparin followed by a moderate dose of warfarin (INR = 2.0-2.5). In one study a moderate dose of heparin (10,000 units subcutaneously twice daily for 16 days) reduced the frequency of arterial embolism (Table 2).

Venous thromboembolism
The risk of clinically diagnosed pulmonary embolism was reduced in all three of the large randomized studies of anticoagulants in acute myocardial infarction. The incidence was reduced from 5.6% to 2.2% in the British Medical Research Council Study ($P < 0.01$) [1], from 6.1% to 3.8% in the Bronx Municipal Centre Study (NS) [2], and from 2.6% to 0.2% in the Veterans Administration Cooperative Trial ($P < 0.005$) [3]. The clinical diagnosis of pulmonary embolism is notoriously unreliable and subject to bias and, therefore, the results of these studies cannot be considered definitive. Nevertheless, the findings of these three studies are supported by autopsy data (Tables 2 and 3) [20-21] and by the results of several studies using ^{125}I-fibrinogen leg scanning to detect venous thrombosis in patients with acute myocardial infarction.

Low dose anticoagulant therapy [31-33] (heparin 5000-7000 units subcutaneously twice daily), as well as full doses of heparin [34-36], appears to be effective in reducing venous thromboembolism in patients with acute myocardial infarction.

Haemorrhagic complications
Haemorrhagic complications were recorded in the 2348 patients who were randomized into anticoagulant therapy in the three large trials [1-3]. Minor bleeding occurred in 7% of patients, major bleeding in 1.5%, central nervous system bleeding in 0.05% and fatal bleeding in none.

Long-term anticoagulant therapy after acute myocardial infarction
Because the risk of death and reinfarction is lower after discharge from hospital, trials of long-term anticoagulant therapy require even larger numbers of patients than the short-term trials to detect true and clinically important differences at conventional levels of statistical significance. None of the earlier studies were large enough to have a reasonable chance of demonstrating a true difference of 20% in death or reinfarction. The three largest trials were the Medical Research Council [9], the Veterans Administration Cooperative Trial [10-11] and the German/Austrian Multi-Centre Clinical Trial [12].

Medical Research Council Trial [9]

This randomized trial included 325 men and 58 women aged 40 to 69 years. Patients were recruited approximately four to six weeks after hospital admission for acute transmural myocardial infarction. Nearly all had received anticoagulant therapy while they were hospitalized before entry into the study. Patients were randomly allocated to receive high-dose anticoagulant therapy (n = 195) or very low doses of phenindione (1 mg) (too small to influence blood coagulation). Over a three-year period of follow-up (Table 4) there was a 30% reduction in the case fatality rate in the treated group (NS). The benefit appeared most marked during the first 6-12 months after hospital discharge. There was a significant reduction in recurrent myocardial infarction [39.9% in control patients compared with 20.5% in the anticoagulant-treated group ($P < 0.001$)]. Thromboembolic episodes (mainly systemic embolism) also occurred significantly less frequently in patients who received full-dose anticoagulants, while haemorrhagic events were significantly more frequent in those receiving full-dose anticoagulants. The haemorrhagic rate in the anticoagulant group was high (41% over three years), but most episodes of bleeding were minor.

Table 4. Effect of long-term anticoagulant therapy on case fatality rates in myocardial infarction

Study	Regimen (no. of patients)	Death	Relative risk reduction (95% confidence limit)	P-value
MRC (*BMJ* 1964)	Control (188) vs	0.213	30%	NS
	AC (195)	0.149	(−6% to 66%)	
German-Austrian (*Ca* 1950)	Control (309) vs	0.10	−18	NS
	AC (320)	0.12	(−65% to 30%)	
VA Coop (*JAMA* 1969)	Control (350) vs	0.326	4.3%	NS
	AC (385)	0.31	(−16% to 25%)	

Veterans Administration Study [10,11]

The study included 747 male patients randomized within 21 days of hospital admission for acute myocardial infarction in 15 Veterans Administration Hospitals. All received anticoagulant therapy during their initial hospital phase and were then randomized to receive either warfarin or placebo after discharge from hospital. The dose of warfarin was adjusted to maintain the prothrombin time (INR 2.0-2.5). The patients were followed for seven years. The mortality rate was significantly less at three years in the group treated with anticoagulant therapy ($P < 0.01$), but at the end of seven years of follow-up the mortality rates were almost identical (42% in the control group and 40% in the anticoagulant-treated group). There was a 25% reduction in the rate of recurrent myocardial infarction in the group treated with anticoagulants (NS). Stroke and other thromboembolic episodes were reported more frequently in the control group ($P < 0.05$).

This clinical trial compared two-year case fatality rates in patients with acute myocardial infarction who were randomly assigned to phenprocoumon (n = 320), acetylsalicylic acid (n = 317) or placebo (n = 309) between 1970 and 1977. Men and women between the ages of 45 and 70 years were recruited within 30 to 42 days after myocardial infarction. The dose of phenprocoumon was adjusted to maintain the thrombotest between 12% and 5% or the prothrombin times between 25% and 15% of control (INR = 2.5-5.0). Patients treated with acetylsalicylic acid received 1.5 g daily, while those patients in the control group received no active drug. There were no significant differences in case fatality rates, fatal or non-fatal recurrent myocardial infarction or in coronary mortality rates, although there were favourable trends in both the case fatality rate and recurrent myocardial infarction in both the aspirin and phenprocoumon groups. There was a non-significant reduction in other thromboembolic complications and a significant increase in haemorrhagic complications in the group treated with phenprocoumon.

The results of the three studies for case fatality rates are summarized in Table 4. Combining the end-points of mortality and recurrent infarction, there was a significant reduction in the Medical Research Council study, due mainly to a reduction in reinfarction and non-significant minimal trends in favour of anticoagulants in the other two studies. There was a reduction in other thromboembolic events in all three studies, and in two this reduction was statistically significant.

The rate of haemorrhagic complications was considerably greater in the patients treated with anticoagulant than in the control group. Most of the haemorrhagic complications were minor and few of the major haemorrhagic complications were fatal. Nevertheless, the side-effects (1% for major haemorrhage), inconvenience and cost of long-term anticoagulant therapy are considerable.

In 1970, an International Anticoagulant Review Group [13] performed an analysis of pooled data from nine controlled, long-term anticoagulant trials involving 2205 men and 282 women. It was concluded that mortality was reduced by 20% in men given long-term anticoagulant, but that the benefit appeared to be restricted to patients with prolonged angina or previous infarction on admission to the trial.

In 1980, the Sixty-Plus Reinfarction Study [37] (Table 5) from The Netherlands, revived the issue of long-term anticoagulant therapy for acute myocardial infarction. Ambulatory patients over 60 years of age from six centres were studied; all were receiving anticoagulants following documented myocardial infarction that had occurred at least six months earlier. This study was designed to determine whether continuation of oral anticoagulant therapy (INR 2.7-4.5) reduces mortality or recurrent infarction. Eligible patients were randomized to continue anticoagulants (439 patients) or to receive placebo (439 patients). A double-blind design was adopted and follow-up was for three years. The data were analyzed both on an intention to treat and on an efficacy basis.

The average age of the patients was 67.6 years; the mean interval since the initial infarction was six years. There was a 55% reduction in the incidence of fatal and non-fatal recurrent myocardial infarction in the group that received anticoagulants. Total deaths and sudden deaths were not significantly different at two years. Although haemorrhagic intracranial events were more frequent in the treated group, non-haemorrhagic intracranial events were reduced in patients who received anticoagulant therapy and there was no significant difference in total intracranial events between the control and the treated groups.

This study demonstrated that continuation of anticoagulant therapy in patients

Table 5. Sixty-plus reinfarction study.

	Placebo	Anticoagulant	P-value
No. of patients	439	439	
Mean age (yr)	67	67	
Time since first infarction (yr)	5	6	
Total deaths within 2 yr	69	51	0.017
Sudden deaths	20	22	
Total intracranial vascular events within 2 yr	20	12	0.16
Haemorrhagic intracranial events	1	9	
Nonhaemorrhagic intracranial events	13	2	
Not identified	6	1	
Total recurrent infarction within 2 yr	64	29	0.0005
Fatal recurrent infarction	27	11	

with a myocardial infarction reduces the incidence of recurrent infarction. The study does not address the questions of efficacy of long-term anticoagulant therapy when commenced soon after myocardial infarction or of their efficacy in patients under 60 years of age.

More recently, the results of a large Norwegian study have been reported confirming the early observations that oral anticoagulants reduce mortality and reinfarction in patients with acute myocardial infarction (unpublished).

Angina

There have been two acceptable trials of anticoagulants in patients with unstable angina.

In 1981, Telford & Wilson [38] performed a randomized study of heparin plus atenolol versus atenolol alone in patients with unstable angina. They reported a marked reduction in mortality and frequency of infarction in patients assigned to heparin plus atenolol. Unfortunately, almost 50% of the 400 patients randomized were not accounted for, so the interpretation of the results remains in doubt.

More recently, Theroux and associates [39] performed a double-blind randomized study comparing heparin (full-dose, intravenous, continuous), aspirin (325 mg twice-daily), heparin plus aspirin and placebo in the treatment of patients with acute unstable angina (Table 6). Major outcome measures were refractory angina, myocardial infarction and death. These were assessed in the first weeks after patient entry to the trial. Both aspirin and heparin reduced the incidence of myocardial infarction and heparin reduced the incidence of refractory angina. The authors concluded that patients with unstable angina should be treated initially with heparin and then with long-term aspirin.

Anticoagulants during or following thrombolytic therapy

The objective of thrombolytic therapy is to restore myocardial perfusion by lysing the obstructing thrombus with minimal delay, and to achieve this goal without producing

Table 6.   Montreal unstable angina study - six day outcome.[+]

Event	Placebo (118)	ASA (121)	Heparin (118)	Heparin and ASA (122)
Refractory angina	27	20	10*	13*
Acute myocardial infarction	14	4*	1*	2*
Death	2	0	0	0
Bleeding** (serious)	6 (2)	4 (2)	10 (2)	10 (4)

[+] Theroux et al. 1988

ASA Acetylsalicylic acid

* $P < 0.05$
** Most bleeding cardiac catheter related

excessive bleeding or promoting re-thrombosis.

Anticoagulants are usually administered after thrombolytic therapy with the aim of reducing the incidence of reinfarction. Anticoagulants are also often administered with tissue plasminogen activator to augment early thrombolysis. Although there is evidence that aspirin reduces the rate of reinfarction [40], there is no reliable information on the effectiveness or lack of effectiveness of anticoagulants in preventing reinfarction following thrombolytic therapy.

Topol and associates [41] reported that early heparin treatment did not influence infarct-related coronary artery patency rates in patients treated with t-PA, but the study was small and lacked the power to exclude a clinically important effect of heparin.

Re-thrombosis after successful coronary thrombolysis occurs in between 5% and 20% of cases [42]. These substantial rates of reocclusion occur despite heparin therapy [43]. Two main contributing factors have been identified for the development of re-thrombosis: persisting severe obstruction and residual thrombosis.

The importance of residual stenosis as a predictor of re-thrombosis has been demonstrated by a number of experimental and clinical studies [44-46]. There is also strong experimental evidence that the presence of a residual thrombus is an important stimulus for re-thrombosis after successful thrombolysis [45,47]. Other evidence suggests that the risk of re-thrombosis increases when the residual thrombosis is seen angiographically after thrombolysis [46,48].

It may be difficult to prevent reocclusion by heparin treatment if there is residual thrombosis after thrombolysis since there is evidence that thrombin which is absorbed to fibrin in a thrombus is relatively resistant to inhibition by heparin [49]. Hirudin and a number of small molecular weight thrombin inhibitors are relatively more effective than heparin in inhibiting fibrin-bound thrombus [49], and these thrombin inhibitors hold promise for preventing re-thrombosis after thrombolytic therapy for coronary artery thrombosis.

References

[1] Report of the Working Party on Anticoagulant Therapy in Coronary Thrombosis to the Medical Research Council. Assessment of short-term anticoagulant administration after cardiac infarction. *Br Med J* 1969; **1**: 335.

[2] Drapkin A, Merskey C. Anticoagulant therapy after acute myocardial infarction: relation of therapeutic benefit to patient's age, sex and severity of infarction. *JAMA* 1972; **222**: 541.

[3] Anticoagulants in acute myocardial infarction. Results of a cooperative clinical trial. *JAMA* 1973; **225**: 724.

[4] Lovell RR, Denborough MA, Nestel PJ, et al. A controlled trial of long-term treatment with anticoagulants after myocardial infarction in 412 male patients. *Med J Aust* 1967; **2**: 97.

[5] MacMillan RL, Brown KW, Watt DL. Long-term anticoagulant therapy after myocardial infarction. *Can Med Assoc J* 1960; **83**: 567.

[6] Meuwissen OJ, Vervoorn AC, Cohen O, et al. Double blind trial of long-term anticoagulant treatment after myocardial infarction. *Acta Med Scand* 1969; **186**: 361.

[7] Conrad LL, Kyriacopoulous JD, Wiggins CW, et al. Prevention of recurrences of myocardial infarction: a double-blind study of the effectiveness of long-term oral anticoagulant therapy. *Arch Intern Med* 1964; **114**: 348.

[8] Wasserman AJ, Gutterman LA, Yoe KR, et al. Anticoagulants in acute myocardial infarction: the failure of anticoagulants to alter mortality in randomized series. *Am Heart J* 1966; **71**: 43.

[9] Second Report of the Working Party on Anticoagulant Therapy in Coronary Thrombosis to the Medical Research Council. An assessment of long-term anticoagulant administration after cardiac infarction. *Br Med J* 1964; **2**: 837.

[10] United States Veterans Administration. Long-term anticoagulant therapy after myocardial infarction. *JAMA* 1965; **193**: 157.

[11] Ebert RV, Borden CV, Hipp HR, et al. Long-term anticoagulant therapy after myocardial infarction: final report of the Veterans Administration Cooperative Study. *JAMA* 1969; **207**: 2263.

[12] Breddin D, Loew D, Lechner K, et al. The German/Austrian Aspirin Trial: a comparison of acetylsalicyclic acid, placebo and phenprocoumon in secondary prevention of myocardial infarction. *Circulation* 1980; **62** (suppl. V): 63.

[13] International Anticoagulant Review Group. Collaborative analysis of long-term anticoagulant administration after acute myocardial infarction. *Lancet* 1970; **i**: 203.

[14] DeWood MA, Spores J, Notske R, et al. Prevalence of total coronary occlusion during the early hours of transmural myocardial infarction. *N Engl J Med* 1980; **303**: 897.

[15] Chalmers TC, Matta RJ, Smith H Jr, et al. Evidence favoring the use of anticoagulants in the hospital phase of acute myocardial infarction. *N Engl J Med* 1977; **297**: 1091.

[16] Wessler S, Cornfield J. Coumarin therapy in acute myocardial infarction: a Hobson's choice. *Arch Intern Med* 1974; **134**: 774.

[17] Modan B, Shani M, Schor S, et al. Reduction of hospital mortality from acute myocardial infarction by anticoagulant therapy. *N Engl J Med* 1975; **292**: 1359.

[18] Tonascia J, Gordis L, Schmerier H. Retrospective evidence favoring use of anticoagulants for myocardial infarction. *N Engl J Med* 1975; **292**: 1362.

[19] Szklo M, Tonascia JA, Goldberg R, et al. Additional data favoring use of anticoagulant therapy in myocardial infarction: a population-based study. *JAMA* 1979; **242**: 1262.

[20] Steffersen KA. Coronary occlusion treated with small doses of heparin. *Acta Med Scand* 1969; **186**: 519.

[21] Hilden T, Iversen K, Raaschou F, et al. Anticoagulants in acute myocardial infarction. *Lancet* 1961; **ii**: 327.

[22] Carleton RA, Sanders CA, Burack WR, et al. Heparin administration after acute myocardial infarction. *N Engl J Med* 1960; **2**: 1002.

[23] Weinreich DJ, Burke JF, Pauletto FJ.
Left ventricular mural thrombi complicating
acute myocardial infarction: long-term
follow-up with serial echocardiography.
Ann Intern Med 1984; **100:** 789.

[24] Ezekowitz MD, Kellerman DJ, Smith EO, et
al.
Detection of active left ventricular
thrombosis during acute myocardial
infarction using indium-III platelet
scintigraphy.
Chest 1984; **86:** 35.

[25] Johannessen KA, Nordrehaug JE, von der
Lippe G.
Left ventricular thrombosis and
cerebrovascular accident in acute
myocardial infarction.
Br Heart J 1984; **51:** 553.

[26] Keating EC, Gross SA, Schlamowitz RA, et
al.
Mural thrombi in myocardial infarctions:
prospective evaluation of two-dimensional
echocardiography.
Am J Med 1983; **74:** 989.

[27] Komrad MS, Coffey CE, Coffey KS, et al.
Myocardial infarction and stroke.
Neurology 1984; **34:** 1403.

[28] Friedman MF, Carlson K, Marcus FI, et al.
Clinical correlations in patients with acute
myocardial infarction and left ventricular
thrombus detected by two-dimensional
echocardiography.
Am J Med 1982; **72:** 894.

[29] Asinger RW, Mikell FL, Elsperger J, et al.
Incidence of left-ventricular thrombosis after
acute transmural myocardial infarction:
serial evaluation by two-dimensional
echocardiography.
N Engl J Med 1981; **305:** 297.

[30] Visser CA, Kan G, Lie KI, et al.
Left-ventricular thrombus following acute
myocardial infarction — a prospective serial
echocardiographic study of 96 patients.
Eur Heart J 1983; **4:** 333.

[31] Marks P, Teather D.
Subcutaneous heparin: a logical prophylaxis
for deep vein thrombosis after myocardial
infarction.
Practitioner 1978; **220:** 425.

[32] Warlow C, Beattie AG, Terry G, et al.
A double-blind trial of low doses of
subcutaneous heparin in the prevention of
deep-vein thrombosis after myocardial
infarction.
Lancet 1973; **ii:** 934.

[33] Handley AJ.
Low-dose heparin after myocardial
infarction.
Lancet 1972; **ii:** 623.

[34] Nicolaides AN, Kakkar VV, Renney JTG, et
al.
Myocardial infarction and deep-vein
thrombosis.
Br Med J 1971; **1:** 432.

[35] Wray R, Maurer B, Shillingford J.
Prophylactic anticoagulant therapy in the
prevention of calf-vein thrombosis after
myocardial infarction.
N Engl J Med 1973; **288:** 815.

[36] Handley AJ, Emerson PA, Fleming PR.
Heparin in the prevention of deep-vein
thrombosis after myocardial infarction.
Br Med J 1972; **2:** 436.

[37] Report of the 60+ Reinfarction Study
Research Group.
A double-blind trial to assess long-term
anticoagulant therapy in elderly patients
after myocardial infarction.
Lancet 1980; **ii:** 989.

[38] Telford AM, Wilson C.
Trials of heparin versus atenolol in
prevention of myocardial infarction in
intermediate coronary syndrome.
Lancet 1981; **i:** 1225.

[39] Theroux P, Ouimet H, McCans J, et al.
Aspirin, heparin, or both to treat acute
unstable angina.
N Engl J Med 1988; **319:** 1105.

[40] ISIS-II Collaborative Group.
Randomized trial of IV streptokinase, oral
aspirin, both, or neither among 17,187 cases
of suspected acute myocardial infarction.
Lancet 1988; **ii:** 349.

[41] Topol EJ, George BS, Kereiakes DJ, et al.
A randomized controlled trial of
intravenous tissue plasminogen activator
and early intravenous heparin in acute
myocardial infarction.
Circulation 1989; **79:** 281.

[42] Sherry S.
Appraisal of various thrombolytic agents in
the treatment of acute myocardial infarction.
Am J Med 1987; **83:** 31.

[43] Williams DO, Borer J, Braunwald E, et al.
Intravenous recombinant tissue type
plasminogen activator in patients with an
acute myocardial infarction. A report from
the NHLBI Thrombolysis in Myocardial
Infarction Trial.
Circulation 1986; **73:** 338.

[44] Badimon L, Badimon JJ, Galvaz A, et al.
Influence of arterial wall damage and wall
stearate on platelet deposition: ex-vivo study
in a swine model.
Atherosclerosis 1986; **6:** 312.

[45] Badimon L, Badimon JJ, Turitto VT, et al.
Mechanisms of arterial thrombosis: platelet
thrombus deposition in areas of stenosis.
Circulation 1987; **76** (suppl. 4): 102.

[46] Gash AK, Spann JS, Sherry S, et al.
Factors influencing reocclusion after
coronary thrombolysis for acute myocardial
infarction.
Am J Cardiol 1986; **57**: 175.

[47] Brown BJ, Gallery CA, Badger RS, et al.
Incomplete lysis of thrombus in the
moderate underlying atherosclerotic lesion
during intracoronary infusion of
streptokinase for acute myocardial
infarction: quantitative angiographic
observations.
Circulation 1986; **73**: 653.

[48] DeGursic P, Theroux P, Bonan R, et al.
Re-thrombosis after successful thrombolysis
and angioplasty in acute myocardial
infarction.
J Am Coll Cardiol 1988; **11**: 192a.

[49] Weitz JI, Hirsh J.
Unpublished observation. (In preparation,
1989.)

5. ADJUVANT STRATEGIES: MECHANICAL INTERVENTIONS

WHAT IS THE NEED FOR ANGIOPLASTY AND SURGERY AFTER THROMBOLYSIS?

G. TOGNONI

The early treatment of patients with acute myocardial infarction with fibrinolytic agents may be considered today the routine management of this clinical condition because of its well-documented efficacy in recanalizing coronary arteries and thereby reducing overall mortality (together with acetylsalicylic acid and possibly beta-blockade). Angioplasty was proposed as a prophylactic treatment in patients with suitable anatomy after fibrinolytic therapy with the aim of reducing reocclusion and recurrent infarctions. Three randomized controlled trials (TAMI, European, TIMI-IIB) testing this approach did not show a reduction in mortality, reinfarction, or both. A 'watchful waiting' approach is suggested by these studies, with the restriction of coronary arteriography and consequent mechanical interventions only to patients with specific clinical indications. This situation has evolved over the last few years as a result of randomized controlled trials. This comprises an interesting reversal of the strategies adopted in various countries, and stimulates a healthy discussion on the relationships between theoretical as opposed to experimental expectations, and controlled clinical results *vis-a-vis* resource allocation.

PTCA AFTER THROMBOLYSIS

A.M. ROSS

Goals of PTCA after thrombolysis
In around 1985, flushed with excitement about the possible impact of intravenous thrombolysis on mortality, it was hoped to add further to these successes with mechanical strategies and adjunctive pharmacologic strategies. The goals that lay behind the addition of mechanical strategies to i.v. lytic therapy are summarized in Table 1.

First, it was thought that reperfusion could be maximized. The outcome/patency rate will vary according to the lytic agent used, but under the very best of circumstances at least 15%-20% of patients will have a persistent occluded artery. Such patients, presumably, will not benefit from interventional therapy unless their vessels can be opened mechanically with an angioplasty.

Second, reocclusion is a serious problem. It is often associated with reinfarction, undoing the benefits of the initial therapy. It was thought that dilating the stenotic segment at the site of the previous thrombus might eliminate reocclusion.

Table 1.

Goals of post-lytic PTCA
Reperfuse lytic failures
Prevent reocclusion
Augment salvage magnitude
Prevent recurrent ischaemia

Third, although the benefit to ventricular function from thrombolysis is easy to demonstrate, the ventricle that is left is rarely a normal one; the myocardium is salvaged, but not all the area that was at risk. A goal of angioplasty was therefore to augment the magnitude of myocardial salvage.

Finally, it was known that after thrombolytic therapy there is a high rate of recurrent ischaemia, cited to be between 10% and 40%. Angioplasty is a tool which is quite effective at dealing with ischaemia due to a dilatable stenosis.

Trials of early PTCA

There have been five randomized trials of early angioplasty versus some other strategy with an eye towards accomplishing these four goals: TAMI, TIMI, the European Cooperative Study Group trial, SWIFT and the Johns Hopkins trial. I will restrict my remarks mostly to the experience with TIMI-IIA and TIMI-IIB.

TIMI-IIA

TIMI-IIA was a trial of just under 400 patients who received tissue-plasminogen activator (t-PA) and were then randomized to receive angiography and angioplasty immediately if technically suitable, or to have the procedure delayed for 24-48 hours. Immediate PTCA was compared to delayed PTCA to determine the impact of the logistical problems involved in transporting patients to a unit able to carry out the proceedure — 12% of tertiary care units in the United States are able to carry out angioplasty.

Comparing the group that had angioplasty at two hours after t-PA therapy to the group that had angioplasty 24-48 hours later, most of the patients in both groups underwent catheterization (Table 2). However, angioplasty was not done in a sizeable fraction of these patients for a variety of reasons. Many of the patients did not have a lesion that was still 60% stenotic at the time of their angiogram; 10%-15% had anatomy judged unsuitable by the operator; although salvage angioplasty was always attempted in patients at two hours, at the time this protocol was written it was assumed that nothing could be gained by salvage angioplasty at 24-48 hours; and in 12% of patients the artery was closed at the time of the delayed angiogram.

When the angioplasty was carried out it was highly successful by common criteria (Table 3). The end-points used were reinfarction, death, and outcome ejection fraction. Using any of these parameters, there was no difference in outcome between the two stategies of immediate and delayed angioplasty, although there seemed to be a trend towards a slightly better outcome with the delayed approach. Also, there was no difference in rates of intracranial bleeding between the two regimens. There was a substantially greater need for blood transfusion in the two hour group. It was therefore concluded that we had chosen well in selecting to compare the less hectic delayed angioplasty to conservative care, and this became the basis of the trial TIMI-IIB.

Table 2. Interventions carried out in patients undergoing immediate or delayed angioplasty.

Interventions	Immediate group (2 h)	Delayed group (18-48 h)
Angio done	99%	81%
PTCA done	73%	65%
No Lesion (<60%)	10%	14%
Unsuitable	16%	8%
Closed	—	12%
Other	1%	1%

Table 3. TIMI-IIA outcome.

	Immediate group	Delayed group
PTCA success	82%	95%
Any complication	12%	4%
Emergency CABG	1%	1%
Outcome ejection fraction	50%	49%
3-week mortality	7.2%	5.7%

TIMI-IIB

Three thousand patients received t-PA, heparin and aspirin, and were then randomized either to the invasive strategy (automatic angiography at 18-24 hours and angioplasty when suitable) or to the conservative strategy (CCU care unless recurrent ischaemia became evident spontaneously or was inducible by exercise test — the appearance of ischaemia triggered selective angiography and angioplasty). The patients entered into this randomization were of typical age, usually male, not-low-risk, 12% were elderly, 13% had prior infarctions, and 50% had anterior infarctions (that is, they were representative of infarct patients as they arrive in the 26 hospitals involved in the trial). Time to treatment was quite early by protocol demand.

Angioplasty in the group assigned to the immediate strategy was actually carried out in only 60% of the patients. It was not undertaken in 13% because the lesion was no longer sufficiently severe to warrant the procedure and it was not undertaken in another 13% because the operator felt it was inadvisable, the most common reasons for that being a left main coronary artery stenosis, a very distal stenosis or very tortuous vessels. Angioplasty was also not carried out owing to the protocol decision that if the infarct artery were still closed at 18-24 hours, salvage angioplasty should not be attempted. When an angioplasty was attempted it was successful by conventional measures in 89% of patients; it was a simple, uncomplicated failure in 4% of patients; and it was a complicated failure in 6%. The complicated failures can be broken down into urgent CABG (2.4%), reinfarction (5.4%) and death (0.5%).

In patients assigned to conservative care, spontaneous or exercise-induced ischaemia led to angioplasty in only 13% of cases by the 14th day and 17% at six weeks.

The primary end-points of this trial were outcome ventricular function, recurrent myocardial infarction and death, with a secondary end-point of exercise-induced ischaemia.

Fig. 1 shows the ejection fractions by radionuclide ventriculograms at the time of hospital discharge;it is evident that there was no difference in global ejection fraction based upon assignment to the invasive or to the conservative strategy. This result is totally consistent with the results of the TAMI trial and the Johns Hopkins trial; the only study of immediate or even delayed angioplasty versus a conservative strategy that has not shown this result is that of Dr Simoons (see page 116). In the TIMI trial, as in the others, there was also a statistically significant more common occurrence of positive exercise tests (almost 18% of those assigned to conservative treatment, less in those who had had an angioplasty). A positive exercise test was, by protocol, an indication to go to angiography and then do an angioplasty or CABG. Since these procedures were generally successful, the conservative strategy group was more like the invasive strategy group when next examined at six weeks.

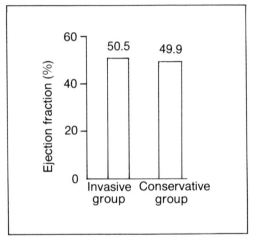

Fig. 1. TIMI-IIB. Left ventricular ejection fraction at the time of hospital discharge.

Fig. 2 shows probably the most important data from TIMI-IIB. In the group of patients who were not thought to be at particularly low risk, the strategy of t-PA, heparin and aspirin was associated with a six-week mortality rate of 5% — there was no difference in that mortality rate based upon assignment to invasive or conservative strategy. There was almost a flat line of survival after 52 weeks. The conclusion of the TIMI investigators was that most patients with acute myocardial infarction could be managed by thrombolytic therapy followed by watchful waiting.

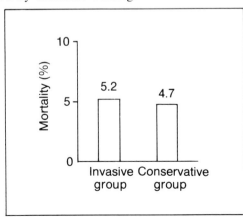

Fig. 2. TIMI-IIB. Six-week mortality rates after myocardial infarction in patients treated by invasive and conservative strategies.

114

Failure to meet the goals of PTCA

The original goals of PTCA after thrombolysis were not achieved, and the question then becomes "Was it because the hypothesis was wrong that dilating the stenotic segment would produce these gains?" or "Was the hypothesis correct but somehow the application incorrect?" I think the answer is some of each.

Part of the hypothesis that dilating the stenotic segment would produce these gains was wrong. Six or eight years ago it was believed that underlying the thrombus was a stenosis >90% in 25% of patients and >75% in another 50% of patients — that is, 75% of patients had a very severe stenosis. That led to the conclusion that the stenosis needed dilating. As the TIMI data show, that is the apparent situation when an angiogram is performed 90 minutes after thrombolytic therapy. However, if the patients are observed over the next few days, it is seen that much of what was thought to be underlying plaque is underlying thrombus which, in most cases, resolves with time. At the 90-minute angiogram in TIMI, the average cross-sectional area of the lumen was 0.7 mm^2, 24 hours later it was 1 mm^2 and 10 days later it was 1-1.5 mm^2 for patients treated with t-PA. Very similar changes were found with patients in TIMI-I treated with streptokinase. These measurements correspond approximately to an 80% stenosis at 90 minutes, 70% the next day, and 60% stenosis at 10 days. So the assumption of the original hypothesis that every patient has a tight stenosis was incorrect.

Part of the application of the technique also has been inadequate. We now know that it is not simple to do acute dilatation in the presence of clot. As reported by Dr Hearse (see page 49), perhaps the most thrombogenic substances in the coronary artery are the intersteces of the thrombus where residual thrombin is bound to fibrin. When a clot is broken open (as with a balloon catheter) a new, tremendously thrombogenic surface is exposed. This may be even more thrombogenic than the subintimal collagen fibres discussed by Dr Fuster (see page 12). As a consequence, acute angioplasty is too often followed by abrupt closures caused by a clotting system that is not adequately paralyzed by heparin and aspirin in conventional doses. There is some distal embolization, and with early interventions the bleeding complications are unavoidable.

The issue of angioplasty to prevent reocclusion and reinfarction seems simple in retrospect. Lysis with t-PA plus heparin and aspirin results in a patency rate of 80%. The late occlusion rate if angioplasty is not performed is 13%, and 15% of patients need an urgent angioplasty if they do not undergo one by protocol on the first day. If angioplasty is performed routinely after successful lysis, about 25% of patients are unsuitable. The incidence of abrupt closure averages 7% when angioplasty is done in successfully opened arteries, and there is an 11% late reocclusion rate — producing an 18% reocclusion rate overall.

Information on salvage angioplasty (dilating those vessels that had not opened with thrombolytic therapy) is fairly consistent: 15% are unsuitable, 15% are failures and there is a 30% late reocclusion rate. When t-PA, heparin and aspirin are given, around 80% of the arteries at zero hours or 90-minutes would be open and 20% would be persistently occluded. If an angioplasty is not performed, two hours later the situation is unchanged. If these patients are restudied at 10 days, there will be approximately 70% with open infarct arteries and 30% with closed arteries due to late reocclusion. If, however, immediate angioplasty is performed on the open arteries after thrombolysis, abrupt occlusion leads to a lower patency rate (71/80) at the end of the two hours. So there is an early loss by dilating those that had been opened by thrombolysis and, since the recurrent occlusion rate over the next week has not been changed by dilating, at seven or 10 days there are fewer open arteries (63/80). When the 20 patients who were closed at the end of t-PA therapy are dilated, the so-called salvage group, the result is 14 open at two hours. However, the reocclusion rate is high over the next 10 days so that the final result is 10 open and 10 closed. Adding together all these results, the aggressive strategy results in 73 open arteries, and the conservative strategy in 70. This is not statistically or clinically significant.

Future developments
What might increase the benefits of post-lytic angioplasty? The first thing that might be improved is patient selection criteria, particularly for the identification of reperfusion failures. Dilation of open vessels will never be of benefit, and if only those who do not open are taken into these aggressive strategies nothing will be lost. Perhaps just as important is the need for fewer PTCA-induced abrupt occlusions. To this end, improved anti-thrombin agents are required and probably better anti-platelet treatments also.

PATIENT SELECTION AND TIMING OF PTCA/CABG AFTER THROMBOLYSIS

M.L. SIMOONS

I wish to provide some data about studies which were not covered in the previous presentation by Dr Ross, present new follow-up data from the European Cooperative Study Group PTCA trial, speculate about the potential role of PTCA, and outline current practice at the Thoraxcenter (University Hospital, Rotterdam) for treating patients after thrombolysis.

A few years ago, it was thought that patency could be increased by immediate PTCA which should lead to further limitation of infarct size and further preservation of left ventricular function. In addition PTCA might prevent recurrent ischaemia, reocclusion and reinfarction, and possibly reduce mortality.

I intend to review four studies comparing thrombolysis with and without PTCA, with different thrombolytic agents: a trial from Mainz by Erbel using intracoronary streptokinase with or without PTCA; the Interuniversity Institute trial with a matched-pair comparison of patients who received PTCA and patients who might have received PTCA if they had been in a suitable hospital; the TAMI trial, and the trial by the European Cooperative Study Group. Patient selection for PTCA was very different between these studies — Erbel and the European Cooperative Study Group elected to attempt PTCA in almost all patients, while the other two performed PTCA in patients with suitable lesions only.

Immediate PTCA
Immediate PTCA after thrombolysis may improve the number of patent vessels, but after 10 to 21 days there was no difference in patency between patients after thrombolysis with intravenous alteplase (rt-PA) plus aspirin and heparin, and similar

therapy plus PTCA (Table 1). Similarly, the other trials did not demonstrate greater patency after PTCA than after thrombolysis. So there is no effect of treatment regimen on the number of patent vessels at the time of discharge. Left ventricular ejection fraction was not different between trials and also mortality was not significantly different. It should be noted that in the trial by Erbel, mortality in both the thrombolysis group and the PTCA group was twice as high as in the other trials although the patient selection criteria were very similar. There was a small improvement in early mortality of the PTCA group in the trial from Mainz, but there was no improvement after PTCA in the other three approaches.

Table 1. Summary of randomized trials comparing i.v. or i.c. thrombolytic therapy (T) without and with immediate angioplasty (PTCA).

Therapy without angioplasty (T)	Treatment including PTCA	Number of patients		Patency (%) after therapy		Patency (%) before discharge		HBDH infarct size		LVEF (%)		Mortality (%)	
		T	PTCA	T	PTCA	T	PTCA	T	PTCA	T	PTCA	T	PTCA
Erbel (Mainz)	i.c. SK + PTCA	79	83	90	86	77	78	—*	—	57	57	16	12
Vermeer (ICIN)	i.c. SK + PTCA	36	36	100	94	86	82	740	760	49	50	5	9
Topol (TAMI)	i.v. rt-PA + PTCA	98	99	100	91	—	—	—	—	56	53	1	4
Simoons (ECSG)	i.v. rt-PA + PTCA	184	183	—	90	90	84	665	706	51	51	3	7

*No data available.

It had been argued that PTCA in the environment of streptokinase would be easier than in the environment of alteplase plus heparin and aspirin, and experience at the Thoraxcenter suggested that there was more immediate rethrombosis when PTCA was performed in the environment of alteplase rather than streptokinase. However, long term follow-up from the Mainz study showed three-year survival to be 80 patients out of 103 patients after thrombolysis without PTCA, and 83 patients out of 103 patients who underwent immediate PTCA. Also the number of patients requiring late bypass surgery was essentially the same. So the streptokinase based study from Mainz did not show any benefit of PTCA on long term survival.

The trials indicate some minor benefits from PTCA in terms of regional wall motion, particularly in a subgroup of patients in the Mainz series, but the evidence is not very convincing.

The conclusion as to the benefit of immediate PTCA is that it does not markedly improve clinical outcome, either in selected patients where the procedure seems feasible or when PTCA is attempted in all patients.

PTCA and residual stenosis
In the trial by the European Cooperative Study Group, PTCA was found to reduce the remaining stenosis but it did not improve the coronary perfusion score (TIMI score). What are the long term implications?

In Table 2, the 14-day one-year follow-up data from this study are presented for the non-invasive group receiving alteplase with heparin and aspirin, and the invasive group receiving the same medication with additional PTCA. There is a further 3% extra mortality in the thrombolysis-only group between 14 days and one year, and also a further 3% mortality in the PTCA group (these figures are similar to those from the TIMI trial where they had 2% extra mortality between six weeks and one year). Also there was 4% extra recurrent infarction and 3% extra recurrent infarction, respectively. There was a greater need for PTCA later on in the thrombolysis-only group. If PTCA has been performed it does not have to be repeated that often. Nevertheless, the number of late PTCAs and the number of patients undergoing surgery are not high, so overall these patients do reasonably well. This is also shown by the New York Heart Association Class grading at one year — the distribution is almost identical between patients receiving alteplase alone and alteplase plus PTCA, with slightly over half of the patients having no symptoms and only 10% with Class 3 or 4 symptoms either due to angina or heart failure.

Table 2.   Follow-up data from patients receiving rt-PA only, or rt-PA and PTCA.

	Mortality (%)		Re-infarction (%)	
	14 day	1 year	14 day	1 year
rt-PA	2.7	5.5	6.0	10.5
rt-PA + PTCA	6.6	9.6	3.8	6.7

Nevertheless, some differences are apparent when patients are grouped according to the status of the infarct vessel at discharge (Table 3). In patients with a total occlusion, or a tight stenosis, both reinfarction and mortality tend to be higher than in patients with a widely patent infarct-related artery at the time of hospital discharge.

Table 3.   Outcome in patients grouped according to status of the infarct-related vessel at hospital discharge.

Diameter stenosis	<50%	51%-90%	91%-100%
n	131	109	75
Mortality	1	4	5
Reinfarction	6	7	5
PTCA/CABG	10	29	15
No event	114	69	50

Medication after treatment was also the same between the two groups. At one year, 13% of patients received anti-coagulants, 50% aspirin, 40% beta-blockers, and 40% calcium-antagonists. It was rare for a patient not to be receiving any medication one year after the procedure. Choice of medication was left to the treating physician.

Rescue PTCA

Rescue PTCA also does not seem to work; that is, reperfusion by mechanical procedure in those patients where thrombolysis fails. Two problems exist. First, it is at present not possible to recognize by non-invasive means those patients in whom thrombolysis fails. New approaches may be developed to allow timely detection of these patients, but at present this is not feasible without angiography. Second, PTCA in occluded vessels in the setting of acute myocardial infarction presents more problems than elective PTCA.

Early PTCA

Early PTCA, studied most extensively by the TIMI Study Group, also appears to be of no advantage. Early PTCA was performed in patients with a patent vessel and a suitable lesion, which amounted to 60% of patients studied after approximately two days. There was no improvement in clinical outcome, as presented by Dr Ross.

Intervention and long-term survival

What might be expected of additional intervention after thrombolytic therapy?Five-year follow-up information from the intracoronary streptokinase trial from the Netherlands showed a further widening in the difference in mortality between the streptokinase treated patients and the conventionally treated patients. There was a 6% difference in mortality after one year increasing to an 8% difference in mortality after five years (Fig. 1). Reinfarction occurred more frequently in streptokinase treated patients, particularly early in the first year. However, after five years there were the same number of reinfarctions — almost one-quarter — in both treatment groups. Additional procedures, surgery and/or PTCA, were performed in patients with recurrent ischaemia. More such procedures were carried out in the streptokinase group; after three months 18% against 14%, slowly increasing over the years until after five years the rate was approximately one-third. Half of the interventions are performed in the first three months and the other half over the subsequent five years.

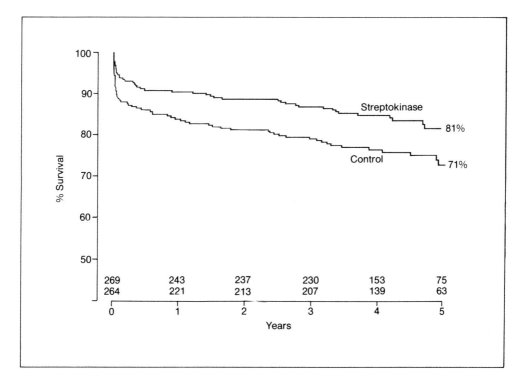

Fig. 1. Survival analysis of all patients allocated to intracoronary streptokinase or conventional therapy (control). The numbers denote patients at risk at the various intervals, streptokinase on top and conventional therapy below. Follow-up was complete at three years. (Reproduced with permission from Simoons ML, Vos J, Tijssen JGP, et al. J Am Coll Cardiol 1989; **14:** 1609–15. [8])

Data were analyzed to determine those factors which might predict long term survival, including all the admission data and data from angiography at hospital discharge. By multivariate analysis it appeared that the best predictor of long term survival was left ventricular function expressed as ejection fraction. The second factor which contributed to long term survival was the residual stenosis of the infarct artery; mortality was greater in patients with a tight stenosis or occlusion than in patients with a more open vessel. A third factor was either the history of previous infarction or the extent of coronary disease. Interestingly, the mode of treatment originally given was not relevant in the long term, suggesting that the effect of thrombolytic therapy is present early on and that afterwards the patients live with the effect that has been achieved. It makes no difference whether the patient has a small infarct which is not treated with thrombolytic therapy or a larger infarct which is reduced by thrombolytic therapy. What matters is the status of the left ventricle and the coronary arteries at the time of hospital discharge.

The relative contribution of the three factors is presented in Fig. 2. Approximately one-quarter of the patients have a poor left ventricular ejection fraction and the remainder have an ejection fraction over 40%. Five-year mortality in hospital survivors was close to 50% in patients with a low ejection fraction, double- or triple-vessel disease and a tight stenosis or occluded infarct-related artery, but was only 4% in patients with a better left ventricular function, single vessel disease and a stenosis < 90%. It appears that in the one-quarter of patients with poor left ventricular function, the best effect that might be expected from revascularization by surgery or PTCA would be a gain in five-year survival of around 10%. In patients with an ejection fraction >40%, the gain would be even smaller.

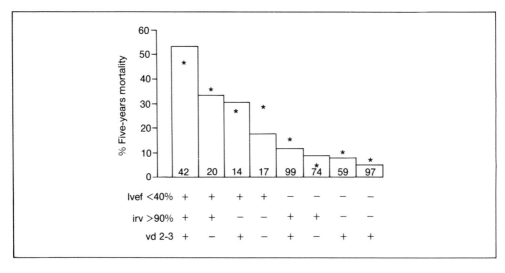

Fig. 2. Prediction of five-year mortality by Cox regression analysis based on left ventricular function, the extent of coronary disease and the status of the infarct-related vessel as assessed at hospital discharge. The height of each bar corresponds with the predicted mortality, and the number in each bar indicates the number of patients in that particular subgroup. The asterixes indicate the actually observed five-year mortality in each subgroup. This analysis was performed in 422 patients with angiography between days 10 and 40. LVEF = left ventricular ejection fraction; IRV >90% = diameter stenosis greater then 90% in the infarct-related vessel; vd 2-3 = patients with double- or triple-vessel coronary disease. (Reproduced with permission from Simoons ML, Vos J, Tijssen JGP, *et al. J Am Coll Cardiol* 1989; **14:** 1609–15. [8])

Current practice

PTCA might become a useful adjunct to thrombolysis provided that the proper patients who require such therapy can be identified and provided that better anti-thrombotic regimens are available at the time of the procedure. At present at the Thoraxcenter, patients with myocardial infarction are treated with alteplase, aspirin and heparin. Patients who develop an infarct during a catheterization procedure are treated with intracoronary streptokinase and, usually, PTCA. In the rare patient in whom thrombolytic therapy is indicated but who has an excessive bleeding risk, we would perform immediate PTCA without thrombolytic therapy. Angiography, PTCA and bypass surgery are performed in three groups of patients. (1) Patients who are admitted with extensive ST-segment elevation who are found to have only a small infarct. Such patients are considered to have a large area at risk for new ischaemia or re-infarction. (2) Patients with recurrent ischaemia post infarction. (3) Patients with angina or ST-segment changes during pre-hospital discharge exercise testing. These three groups amount to about one-quarter or at most one-half of the patients after myocardial infarction.

References

[1] Erbel R, Pop T, Henrichs KJ, et al. Percutaneous transluminal coronary angioplasty after thrombolytic therapy: a prospective controlled randomized trial. J Am Coll Cardiol 1986; **8**: 485–95.

[2] Erbel R, Pop T, Diefenbach C, et al. Long-term results of thrombolytic therapy with and without percutaneous transluminal coronary angioplasty. J Am Coll Cardiol 1989; **14**: 276–85.

[3] Topol EJ, Califf RM, George BS, et al. and the TAMI Study Group. A randomized trial of immediate versus delayed elective angioplasty after intravenous tissue plasminogen activator in acute myocardial infarction. N Engl J Med 1987; **317**: 581–9.

[4] Vermeer F, Simoons ML, de Feyter PJ, et al. Immediate PTCA after successful thrombolysis with intracoronary streptokinase, three years follow up. Eur Heart J 1988; **9**: 346–53.

[5] Simoons ML, Arnold AER, Betriu A, et al. Thrombolysis with tissue plasminogen activator in acute myocardial infarction: no additional benefit from immediate percutaneous coronary angioplasty. Lancet 1988; **i:** 197–203.

[6] TIMI-IIA. Immediate vs delayed catheterization and angioplasty following thrombolytic therapy for acute myocardial infarction. JAMA 1988; **260**: 2849–58.

[7] TIMI-IIB. Comparison of invasive and conservative strategies after treatment with intravenous tissue plasminogen activator in acute myocardial infarction. N Engl J Med 1989; **320**: 618–27.

[8] Simoons ML, Vos J, Tijssen JGP, et al. Long-term benefit of early thrombolytic therapy in patients with acute myocardial infarction: 5 year follow up of a trial conducted by the Interuniversity Cardiology Institute of the Netherlands. J Am Coll Cardiol 1989; **14**: 1609–15.

[9] Arnold AER, Werf F van der, Simoons ML, et al. One year follow up of the rt-PA/placebo and the rt-PA/PTCA trial of the European Cooperative Study Group. Submitted for publication.

6. THE FUTURE

NEW DEVELOPMENTS IN THROMBOLYTIC THERAPY

D. COLLEN

Introduction

The immediate goal of thrombolytic therapy is the recanalization of occluded coronary arteries. This should be achieved as effectively, quickly and selectively as possible. At present these goals have not been reached and therefore there is potential for further improvement. Two major approaches to increasing the efficacy, speed and selectivity of thrombolytic agents are being pursued. Either the fibrin dissolving potency of thrombolytic agents can be increased or, alternatively, strategies can be designed aimed at dispersing platelet-rich thrombi [1]. These two approaches may in fact be complementary, as suggested by pre-clinical research evidence.

Thrombolytic therapy in acute myocardial infarction

Compared to the first-generation thrombolytic agents such as streptokinase and urokinase, it was hoped, based on their biochemical properties, that the fibrin-specific agents tissue-type plasminogen activator (t-PA) and single chain urokinase-type plasminogen activator (scu-PA, prourokinase) would be more effective and more specific. Table 1 summarizes the results of the two randomized studies available which directly compare the efficacy of streptokinase and t-PA, the TIMI-I trial [2] and the European Cooperative Study Group trial [3]. Meta-analysis of the results from the two trials was performed by Chesebro *et al.* [4]; the 90-minute patency rate was 70% with t-PA and 46% with streptokinase (ratio 1.52, P-value 0.001).

Table 1. Coronary artery patency after thrombolysis with streptokinase (SK) or rt-PA in randomised trials (data from Chesebro *et al.*, 1988).

Time from onset of symptoms to therapy	rt-PA	SK	P-value
Less than 3h			
ESCG	23/29 (79%)	20/35 (57%)	0.06
TIMI	11/13 (85%)	11/21 (52%)	0.06
Combined	34/42 (81%)	31/56 (55%)	<0.01
3 to 6h			
ECSG	20/32 (62%)	14/26 (54%)	NS
TIMI	89/130 (69%)	50/125 (40%)	<0.001
Combined	109/162 (67%)	64/151 (42%)	<0.001
Overall			
ECSG	43/61 (70%)	34/61 (56%)	<0.06
TIMI	100/143 (70%)	61/146 (42%)	<0.001
Combined	143/204 (70%)	92/207 (46%)	<0.001

When patency data from non-comparative trials with similar end-points (angiography around 90 minutes) are pooled, patency rates of 48% and 75% for streptokinase and t-PA, respectively, are obtained [5]. If the results from the recent PRIMI-trial [6] are included (streptokinase associated with 64% reperfusion at 90 minutes), the pooled value for streptokinase rises to 51%. When true reperfusion data (at 90-minute angiography) are evaluated, the efficacy is slightly lower — 42% reperfused with streptokinase and 67% with t-PA [5]. These data indicate that in terms of early reperfusion, t-PA is a better agent than streptokinase. It is, however, possible that late reopening is also beneficial. Nevertheless, in-hospital mortality has been consistently higher in patients with an occluded artery at 90 minutes than in patients with early recanalization of the artery.

Given that the efficient early opening of an artery is important for survival, why is there as yet no proof that the difference in efficacy between agents is associated with better ventricular function or mortality? This may be because the studies carried out so far do not have the required statistical power to reach levels of significance. Indeed, to show that a difference in efficacy of 50% patency with streptokinase versus 75% with t-PA translates into a significant difference in ejection fraction, and assuming that preservation of left ventricular function is directly proportional to efficacy for early coronary thrombolysis, over 800 patients would be required in a single randomized study. The reasoning behind these numbers is outlined elsewhere [7]. Of the most recent studies comparing the effect of streptokinase and rt-PA on left ventricular function, Dr Norris (see page 76) has shown no difference. Magnani and coworkers [8] studied 171 patients, of whom seven patients treated with streptokinase and four patients treated with rt-PA died early. A significantly better ejection fraction was found in the rt-PA group as determined by echocardiography (56% *vs.* 51%, $P = 0.05$) and a statistically non-significant effect by contrast ventriculography (55% *vs.* 53%, $P =$ NS).

Furthermore, trials using ejection fraction as an end-point have been unable to show good correlation between improvement of ejection fraction and reduction of early mortality [9]. None of the placebo-controlled trials in which the active treatment group received streptokinase, t-PA or APSAC, showed a significant difference for both ejection fraction and mortality.

Simoons compiled mortality data from placebo-controlled trials of intra-coronary/intravenous streptokinase, APSAC and t-PA [10]. There was no significant difference between the reduction in mortality obtained with streptokinase and t-PA. Again, these trials do not have sufficient statistical power to prove that the outcome and the effect on mortality is proportional to efficacy. To show, in a comparative trial, a 50% difference in the reduction of mortality between streptokinase and t-PA (that is, respective mortality rates of 6.75% and 5.6% based on a control mortality of 9% and a reduction by streptokinase of 25%), 11,800 patients would have to be enrolled [7]. Until such a trial is carried out, data presently available neither support nor disprove the hypothesis that efficacy for early coronary thrombolysis determines outcome.

New trends in thrombolytic therapy

It has been possible to increase the efficacy of thrombolytic agents to some extent although the clinical benefit remains to be confirmed. The administration schemes may also be improved. The standard dose of streptokinase is 1.5 million units over one hour. However, this may not be the optimal dose and changing the dosage may lead to increased efficacy. The situation for t-PA is less clear. There is some preliminary data that t-PA may work as a bolus injection, or that it may be given in cocktails. In one study from the United States, the combination of low dose t-PA and full dose streptokinase achieved surprisingly good results. Thus, optimizing the dose of a thrombolytic agent may improve efficacy.

Improving fibrin-dissolving potency

Present research in this area is being carried out along several lines.

Synergism

Several synergistic combinations of thrombolytic agents have been tried. At the Center for Thrombosis and Vascular Research (Leuven), 19 patients were given single chain t-PA and scu-PA in combination at around one-third to one-quarter of the therapeutic doses; a 70% reperfusion rate was obtained (unpublished results). Thus synergistic combinations may reduce the total amount of agent required, and with these combined low doses there may be no fibrinogen breakdown and, potentially, reduced bleeding tendency.

Mutants of t-PA and scu-PA

Improvements in efficacy have been attempted through modification of existing agents by recombinant DNA technology, and also through the development of artificial molecules. For example, t-PA is cleared from the blood very rapidly via a high affinity mechanism in the liver. If that recognition signal could be eliminated, the resulting t-PA molecule could have a prolonged half-life. Such deletion mutants have been produced by deletion of the finger and growth factor domains in t-PA and have been shown to have a five-fold longer half-life and a ten-fold lower clearance in the dog [11].

In the pharmaceutical industry, much work is being carried out on mutants; around 60 patent applications covering t-PA mutants appear to have been submitted in the European patent office in Munich.

Chimers of t-PA and scu-PA

Another approach is the construction of chimeric molecules, in which different natural molecules are joined together by recombinant DNA technology. For example, the scu-PA molecule has no affinity for fibrin although it has significant fibrin specificity and it is not neutralized by inhibitors in the blood. Efforts are being undertaken to combine this natural molecule with a delivery system to the fibrin molecule. First attempts have involved attachment of scu-PA to the amino-terminal part of t-PA, which is responsible for t-PA's fibrin affinity [12]. Unfortunately, although this chimer has a higher fibrin affinity than scu-PA, its affinity is not as high as that of t-PA, whilst its thrombolytic potency has remained at the level of the scu-PA molecule [13]. The chimeric approach remains promising, however, since it may enable the development of an agent that has increased fibrin selectivity at reduced dose.

Antibody-targeted therapy

The action of thrombolytic agents may be targeted towards the thrombus with the use of fibrin-specific antibodies. Haber *et al.* [14] obtained a targeting effect of around four-fold. At the Center for Thrombosis and Vascular Research (Leuven), a conjugate of recombinant scu-PA with a murine monoclonal antibody directed against fibrin fragment D-dimer has been developed with an eight-fold higher thrombolytic patency than scu-PA in a rabbit jugular vein thrombosis model [15].

Interfering with platelet-rich thrombus
This may be achieved by platelet disaggregation and prevention of platelet re-aggregation. High local concentrations of thrombolytic agents can disperse platelet aggregates; hence, intracoronary administration is more effective in some cases. The thrombolytic agent may be combined with an anti-platelet agent to improve efficacy, as has been clinically suggested for the combination of aspirin with streptokinase in the ISIS-II study [16]. The plasminogen activator may also be targeted to platelet aggregates with monoclonal antibodies.

A problem delaying the development of strategies directed against the platelet-rich thrombus has been, hitherto, the unavailability of any suitable animal models. However, in Boston a dog model has now been developed [17] in which t-PA boluses were shown to act against erythrocyte-rich clots, but reocclusion by platelet rich thrombus occurred consistently. When, however, t-PA was administered with anti-platelet antibody, rapid reperfusion without reocclusion was consistently observed [18].

Reducing the bleeding tendency
A major problem with thrombolytic agents is the need to distinguish between haemostatic clot and occlusive thrombus. There is some evidence that this may be possible. A recent study with recombinant t-PA in 50 patients with acute myocardial infarction showed that bleeding times remained normal throughout the infusion period in 60% of patients, indicating significant discrimination between haemostatic plugs and occlusive thrombi [19].

Bleeding times may serve as a useful research parameter in attempts to improve thrombolytic regimens. In Leuven, rabbits were given aspirin, t-PA and plasminogen activator inhibitors [20]. Aspirin or t-PA also marginally prolonged bleeding times, but when administered together bleeding time was significantly increased. Administration of the plasminogen activator inhibitor-1 resulted in immediate normalization of the bleeding time, which is indicative of interactive effects between antiplatelet agents and thrombolytic agents.

Conclusion
Pharmacological coronary artery reperfusion early during acute myocardial infarction improves outcome although there is some evidence that late reperfusion may also be of benefit. Fibrin-specific agents may have limited maximal efficacy. A certain percentage of patients with highly platelet-rich clots may be intrinsically resistant to even the best thrombolytic agents, and therefore 100% efficacy may never be achieved using fibrin-resolving agents alone. However, in some of these patients the co-administration of agents dispersing aggregated platelets may improve the outcome. The mechanism of bleeding remains to be further explored. Most likely more effective agents, better strategies and improved outcome will become available for patients with myocardial infarction.

References

[1] Collen D, Gold HK.
Fibrin-specific thrombolytic agents and new approaches to coronary arterial thrombolysis. In: Julian D, Kübler W, Norris RM, Swan HJC, Collen D, Verstraete M, eds. *Thrombolysis in cardiovascular disease.* Basel: Marcel Dekker Inc., 1989; 45–67.

[2] TIMI Study Group.
The Thrombolysis in Myocardial Infarction (TIMI) trial: phase I findings. *N Engl J Med* 1985; **312:** 932–6.

[3] Verstraete M, Bernard R, Bory M, *et al.*
Randomised trial of intravenous recombinant tissue-type plasminogen

activator versus intravenous streptokinase in acute myocardial infarction.
Lancet 1985; **i:** 842–7.

[4] Chesebro JH, Knatterud G, Braunwald E.
Thrombolytic therapy. [Correspondence]
N Engl J Med 1988; **319:** 1544–5.

[5] Collen D, Lijnen HR, Todd PA, Goa KL.
Tissue-type plasminogen activator. A review of its pharmacology and therapeutic use as a thrombolytic agent.
Drugs 1989; **38:** 346–88.

[6] PRIMI Trial Study Group.
Randomised double-blind trial of recombinant pro-urokinase against streptokinase in acute myocardial infarction.
Lancet 1989; **i:** 863–8.

[7] Collen D.
Coronary thrombolysis: streptokinase or recombinant tissue-type plasminogen activator (rt-PA)?
Ann Int Med 1990; **112:** 529–38.

[8] Magnani B, Plasminogen Activator Italian Multicenter Study (PAIMS) Group.
Comparison of intravenous recombinant single chain human tissue-type plasminogen activator (rt-PA) with intravenous streptokinase in acute myocardial infarction.
J Am Coll Cardiol 1989; **13:** 19–26.

[9] Van de Werf F.
Discrepancies between the effects of coronary reperfusion on survival and left ventricular function.
Lancet 1989; **i:** 1367–8.

[10] Simoons ML.
Trials with rt-PA in acute myocardial infarction. In: Julian D, Kübler W, Norris RM, Swan HJC, Collen D, Verstraete M, eds. *Thrombolysis in cardiovascular disease.* Basel: Marcel Dekker Inc., 1989; 87–102.

[11] Cambier P, Van de Werf F, Larsen GR, Collen D.
Pharmacokinetics and thrombolytic properties of a nonglycosylated mutant of human tissue-type plasminogen activator, lacking the finger and growth factor domains, in dogs with copper coil-induced coronary artery thrombosis.
J Cardiovasc Pharmacol 1988; **11:** 468–72.

[12] Nelles L, Lijnen HR, Collen D, Holmes WE.
Characterization of a fusion protein consisting of amino acids 1 to 263 of tissue-type plasminogen activator and amino acids 144 to 411 of urokinase-type plasminogen activator.
J Biol Chem 1987; **262:** 10855–62.

[13] Collen D, Stassen JM, Demarsin E, Kieckens L, Lijnen HR, Nelles L.
Pharmacokinetic and thrombolytic properties of chimaeric plasminogen activators consisting of the NH_2-terminal

region of human tissue-type plasminogen activator and the COOH-terminal region of human single chain urokinase-type plasminogen activator.
J Vasc Med Biol 1989; **1:** 234–40.

[14] Haber E, Quertermous T, Matsueda GR, Runge MS.
Innovative approaches to plasminogen activator therapy.
Science 1989; **243:** 51–6.

[15] Collen D, Dewerchin M, Stassen JM, Kieckens L, Lijnen HR.
Thrombolytic and pharmacokinetic properties of conjugates of urokinase-type plasminogen activator with a monoclonal antibody specific for cross-linked fibrin.
Fibrinolysis 1989; **3:** 197–202.

[16] ISIS-2 (Second International Study of Infarct Survival) Collaborative Group.
Randomised trial of intravenous streptokinase, oral aspirin, both, or neither among 17,187 cases of suspected acute myocardial infarction: ISIS-2.
Lancet 1988; **ii:** 349–60.

[17] Yasuda T, Gold HK, Fallon JT, *et al.*
A canine model of coronary artery thrombosis with superimposed high grade stenosis for the investigation of rethrombosis after thrombolysis.
J Am Coll Cardiol 1989; **13:** 1409–14.

[18] Yasuda T, Gold HK, Leinbach RC, *et al.*
Tissue plasminogen activator (t-PA) resistant platelet rich white thrombus (WT) and combination treatment of t-PA and antiplatelet antibody to GPIIb/IIIa receptor (7E3). [Abstract 0058]
Circulation 1988; **78:** II-15.

[19] Gimple LW, Gold HK, Leinbach RC, *et al.*
Correlation between template bleeding times and spontaneous bleeding during treatment of acute myocardial infarction with recombinant tissue-type plasminogen activator.
Circulation 1989; **80:** 581–8.

[20] Vaughan DE, Declerck PJ, De Mol M, Collen D.
Recombinant plasminogen activator inhibitor-1 reverses the bleeding tendency associated with combined administration of tissue-type plasminogen activator and aspirin in rabbits.
J Clin Invest 1989; **84:** 586–91.

THE LOGISTICS OF PRE-HOSPITAL CARE FOR ACUTE MYOCARDIAL INFARCTIONS

A. LEIZOROVICZ

The treatment at home by mobile coronary care units of patients with myocardial infarction is not new. In the mid-1960s several organizations, especially in the UK, were set up to treat patients at home, and several studies have evaluated the benefits from this kind of early intervention. One of the conclusions of these studies is that the decision whether a mobile coronary care unit is of value to a community must be based upon its success with the patients it treats, its success in reaching patients in need, and the resources available.

Data from hospital thrombolytic trials have shown that the earlier treatment is administered, the better the outcome. Fig. 1 shows the reduction in mortality related to interval from symptom onset to treatment in the ISIS-II trial. Obviously, any system that can reduce the time to intervention by treating patients at home is of potential interest. What are the logistical implications of this kind of intervention, in terms of organization, personnel, equipment, and so on.

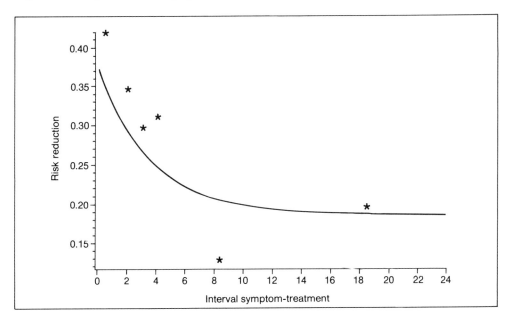

Fig. 1. Risk reduction in vascular deaths in patients treated with streptokinase versus placebo. Modelled from ISIS-II.

Mobile coronary care units

Having been in contact directly or indirectly with many mobile coronary care units or their equivalent, I believe there is no such thing as a standard model for a mobile coronary care unit. On the contrary, these systems are very differently organized, staffed and equipped, not only from one country to another but even from one city to another within one country. In Lyon, patients dial 15 (the national telephone number in

France for any kind of medical emergency). The operator switches the call to an emergency control point where two doctors are in attendance. These doctors will have been involved in the emergency system for at least three years and they can decide upon the appropriate intervention. If they suspect a myocardial infarction, they could decide to send a team consisting of a driver trained in cardiopulmonary resuscitation, a nurse and a doctor. On arrival at the home, the patient is examined, an ECG can be performed, and if the diagnosis is myocardial infarction, a thrombolytic may be injected. When the patient is stabilized, he is moved to the nearest hospital in the ambulance/mobile, which is equipped with oxygen, a defibrillator and several drugs. Also there is a telephone so that a bed may be reserved at the hospital while the patient is being transported.

This is only one example of what is available in France, and it is different from practice in other countries. It is not possible to give here a comprehensive review of all the different logistics which have been adopted in various countries; whether by a national organization as in France, Belgium or the USSR, or by local organizations as in most other countries. What is mportant is that the calls for help should be centralized and that a unique national number can be assigned rather than to have several confidential telephone numbers; it is also important that these numbers are available to the public and not only to the general practitioner.

Although this presentation has been referring to mobile coronary care units, such units are the exception rather than the rule. In most cases, the emergency units are polyfunctional mobile rescue units which can intervene for any medical emergency. Sometimes the unit may be manned by the fire department, as in Paris. Whether the unit is hospital-based or non-hospital-based does not matter as long as the personnel are fully trained, and some units are even run by private organizations. Two of the most important aspects of pre-hospital care are the notification and education of the public, and the way this is integrated with the general health organization and with the general practitioner and cardiologist. There has to be a very good interaction between these two — the emergency service should be known and trusted by the public and also by the general practitioners and cardiologists.

Personnel

For legal reasons in most countries a doctor has to be present to prescibe a drug. Cardiologists are rarely seen in mobile coronary care units; internists are sometimes present and, in most cases, an anaesthesiologist or resident. Whether these doctors are especially dedicated to mobile coronary care units or whether they are just chosen at the hospital when there is a call, differs from one city to another. There are also trained nurses and paramedics — well-trained paramedics in some units, especially in England. Probably the nurses and paramedics are as capable as many doctors in the diagnosis of myocardial infarction and in Sweden nurses are allowed to treat patients; this would be valuable for intervention in myocardial infarction patients. At the emergency control point it is necessary to have a reliable pair of people who could detect the need for an emergency unit to be dispatched, and whether these are doctors or firemen they would have to be trained carefully.

Equipment

Requirements are a van or car (sometimes even an helicopter), an electrocardiogram (ECG) recorder, monitors, defibrillators, oxygen supply, and appropriate medications. In terms of the ECG, a simple recorder would, in most cases, suffice to make a diagnosis of myocardial infarction. Some units are equipped with interpretative/

integrated ECG recorders that might be useful. There is discussion as to whether there is a need for transmission of the ECG — my suspicion is that, in most cases, it is not necessary if the personnel in the ambulances are fully trained. Thus the loss of time to transmit the ECG may be avoided. A collaborative survey [1] was carried out of 2,254 patients with chest pain from several cities in Europe, to determine the value of the first ECG, whether recorded in a mobile coronary care unit or in hospital. It was found that wherever the first ECG was performed, when the first ECG was labelled positive (that is, it showed ST-elevation), in more than 80% of the cases, diagnosis of myocardial infarction could be made accurately; when the first ECG appeared negative by this criterion, in 30% of the cases there was later confirmation of myocardial infarction (Fig. 2). The value of the first ECG with respect to prognosis was also the same whether taken in hospital or a mobile coronary care unit.

Ventricular fibrillation is a major concern in patients with myocardial infarction. However, ISIS-II showed that there was no excess of ventricular fibrillation in patients treated with thrombolytics, and possibly even a reduced incidence of ventricular fibrillation. So whether there is a need for a defibrillator in the mobile coronary care unit might be questioned; however, in most instances there are defibrillators. There are also drugs which are available to treat complications.

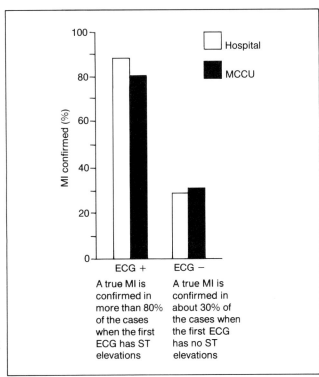

Fig. 2. Confirmed myocardial infarctions and first ECG findings.

Patient selection

Which patients can be treated at home?In France, about one-third to one-half of patients hospitalized for myocardial infarction are eligible for thrombolysis, and only one-tenth of all the hospitalized patients would be eligible for home thrombolysis. Only one-third of all hospitalized patients are retrieved by a mobile coronary care unit, and about 1% of patients seen by the mobile units do not reach the hospital — possibly they die before arrival. However, large differences exist between cities in the proportion of myocardial infarction patients transported by the mobile coronary care units. This depends largely on the implementation and reputation in the city, as well as on the availability of alternative systems.

It is important to evaluate the time gained with home treatment. The preliminary experience of EMIP shows there is about a one-hour gain between the first possibility to inject a treatment at home and the same injection in the hospital. However, such studies might be biased because the fact that the diagnosis has been already made at home reduces delay within the hospital.

Conclusion

A lot of questions remain to be answered about pre-hospital thrombolysis. Is there always a gain in time? Does this translate into a gain in life? What are the important areas of diagnosis, the adequate management of complications at home, the merits of the different types of mobile units, benefit:risk ratios for patients retrieved by mobile coronary care units, and the cost:benefit ratios. Answers to these questions can only be provided by randomized trials. At present, on the one hand some units already routinely treat patients with thrombolytic therapy at home (in Berlin, Jerusalem, Marseille and so on) and, on the other hand, there are people who say it is useless and even dangerous to do so. Who is correct?

The European Myocardial Infarction Project has just been set up to determine the risk:benefit ratio of treating patients at home with anistreplase (APSAC) and also to evaluate the diagnostic criteria which will be used for including the patients. The different ways patients are treated and the logistical aspects will also be recorded. Patients who are treatable include patients with typical chest pain and either typical ECG involving ST-elevation or patients with atypical ECG but strong history of coronary heart disease. Patients will receive either anistreplase at home and placebo in the hospital or placebo at home and anistreplase in the hospital. The patients will be followed up after discharge from the hospital for long-term survival. The study will involve several countries in Europe and possibly also Canada. The present objective is to recruit more than 10,000 patients and so far about 600 patients have been included.

References

[1] Report of the European Myocardial Infarction Project (EMIP) Sub-Committee. Potential time saving with pre-hospital intervention in acute myocardial infarction. *Eur Heart J* 1988; **9**: 118–24.

STRATEGIES AND PROBLEMS IN PRE-HOSPITAL TREATMENT IN ACUTE MYOCARDIAL ISCHAEMIA

S. HOLMBERG

Two studies have been performed in Gothenburg that illustrate possible strategies and specific problems in prehospital care. The first study was a mass media campaign. The second was the TEAHAT study which evaluates thrombolytic therapy given either in the prehospital phase or in hospital.

In Gothenburg patients with chest pain rarely call general practitioners. Patients either go directly to the emergency room of one of the two hospitals or they call for an ambulance to transport them to hospital. Only the latter group can be identified for prehospital treatment.

The first study was a mass media campaign to reduce delay time between onset of chest pain and medical treatment and to increase the use of ambulances in patients with suspected myocardial infarction [1]. The campaign was known as HJÄRTA-SMÄRTA-90,000, a rhythmic sounding name in the Swedish language. The direct translation would be HEART-PAIN-90,000; 90,000 being the national phone number for emergency calls. The message was 'chest pain of more than 15 minutes duration might indicate acute myocardial infarction and requires immediate hospitalization. Call for an ambulance!'. The message was spread via posters, leaflets, articles in newspapers and advertisements. The campaign was run for one year, with a high intensity campaign in the first month and repeated campaign activities approximately once a month thereafter.

The TEAHAT study was a randomized placebo-controlled study of the effect of rt-PA given in the prehospital phase or in hospital [2]. Maximal effort was exerted to identify all patients with myocardial infarction in Gothenburg and to start treatment early — if possible in the prehospital period. The inclusion criteria were age below 65 years and chest pain of more than 15 minutes but less than 2 hours and 45 minutes duration. No ECG criteria were required. During the study period 479 patients were available for evaluation. Of the 145 available in the prehospital phase, 44 had exclusion criteria and 101 were included and randomized (that is, 29% of the 352 included patients).

Early identification
Even the high intensity media campaign failed to increase the proportion of patients calling for an ambulance. During the control period of the two years preceding the study, 61% of patients with chest pain called for an ambulance. After the first four months of the campaign 64% called for an ambulance, and after one year the figure was 63%.

Early access to the patient
The media campaign resulted in a significant shortening of delay time to hospitalization or to treatment. During the two year control period before the campaign, the median delay time from start of symptoms to arrival in hospital was three hours. During the first four months of the campaign there was a significant reduction of delay time down to two hours for patients with acute myocardial infarction coming to hospital. For all patients with acute myocardial infarction during the first year of the campaign, the median delay time from start of symptoms to arrival in hospital was 2 hours and 20 minutes — a reduction in delay time of 40 minutes.

In the 101 patients treated in the prehospital phase, the shortening of delay time from start of symptoms to start of treatment was 40 minutes. This reduction in delay time was the result of start of treatment outside hospital.

Thus, patients could be reached earlier for start of treatment both because patients came earlier to hospital after start of symptoms and because patients could be identified for start of treatment outside hospital.

Selection of patients

Prehospital treatment accentuates the problems associated with the proper selection of patients. During the TEAHAT study the ambulance dispatchers suspected myocardial infarction in 350 of the emergency calls. To all these cases a paramedic ambulance was dispatched with a cardiologist added to the regular crew. The inclusion in the TEAHAT study was based on strong clinical suspicion of myocardial infarction without ECG criteria.

Among the 350 cases, the cardiologist had a suspicion of myocardial infarction in 145 while in 205 patients he had not. Of these 205 patients, 13 actually developed a myocardial infarction and in 11 of these there were contraindications to thrombolysis. Thus only two patients in this group were excluded from active therapy. Among the 145 patients where the cardiologist suspected myocardial infarction, only 59 actually developed myocardial infarction. Thus, only in 59 of 350 (17%) cases where the ambulance dispatchers suspected myocardial infarction was the diagnosis confirmed (Table 1).

Table 1. Prehospital selection of patients. Final diagnosis of 350 patients where ambulance dispatchers suspected myocardial infarction.

	'90,000' calls	
AMI suspected by ambulance dispatchers (chest pain <3 h)	350	
Clinical diagnosis by cardiologist in ambulance (no ECG criteria)	145 (41%) AMI suspected	205 (59%) AMI not suspected
Definite AMI	59 (17%)	13 (4%)

It is interesting to analyse the importance of ECG changes for the prediction of myocardial infarction. In the TEAHAT study an ECG was taken immediately after start of treatment. Of the 352 patients included in the study, 200 had ST-elevation of 2 mm or more in at least two ECG leads. Of those, 177 (88%) developed acute myocardial infarction. On the other hand, in the remaining 152 cases only 21% developed myocardial infarction (Table 2). These data, together with the demonstrated low precision of clinical diagnosis in prehospital patients, strongly suggest that ECG criteria should be used for selection of patients. This is especially important in the prehospital period when time is limited and, for technical reasons, it is often difficult to make a detailed analysis of symptoms and signs.

Conclusion

In Gothenburg, two-thirds of patients with myocardial infarction call for an ambulance and could thus theoretically be identified for prehospital treatment. In reality less than one-third were included for treatment in the TEAHAT study because of the inclusion and exclusion criteria used.

Ambulance dispatchers had a low specificity in selecting patients with suspected

Table 2. Diagnosis in relation to ECG.

	Patients with ST-elevation	Patients without ST-elevation
AMI suspected by cardiologist	200	152
Definite AMI	177	32
% definite AMI	88	21

myocardial infarction for prehospital treatment.

A high intensity mass media campaign did not increase the proportion of patients with acute myocardial infarction calling for an ambulance.

The campaign significantly shortened the delay time from start of symptoms to start of treatment.

In patients where thrombolytic therapy was started in the prehospital phase, the delay time from start of symptoms to start of treatment was shortened by 40 minutes.

Patient selection for thrombolytic therapy should, especially in the prehospital period, be based on ECG criteria.

References

[1] Herlitz J, Hartford M, Blohm M, et al. Effect of a media campaign on delay times and ambulance use in suspected acute myocardial infarction. *Am J Cardiol* 1989; **64**: 90–3.

[2] TEAHAT Study Group. Very early thrombolytic therapy in suspected acute myocardial infarction. *Am J Cardiol* (in press).

PRE-HOSPITAL MANAGEMENT OF ACUTE MYOCARDIAL INFARCTION: PATIENT AND GENERAL PRACTITIONER INTERACTIONS

R.G. WILCOX, J.M. ROWLEY

Introduction

There is no doubt that a rapid response strategy is necessary for patients who have sudden collapse out-of-hospital, particularly since new thrombolytic treatments offer the very real possibility that we can ameliorate the effects of acute myocardial infarction and improve outcome [1-4]. Some studies indicate that if patients can be treated particularly quickly, for example within one hour of symptom onset, the most remarkable reduction in death may be obtained. However, even in the GISSI trial only about 11% of the patients actually received thrombolytic treatment within one hour of onset of symptoms [1].

Many factors determine how long it takes a patient to arrive in a hospital coronary care unit after the onset of major symptoms. These times have been assessed in Nottingham over the period of the last five years and are comparable to results obtained by other units taking part in our multi-centre studies in acute myocardial infarction. In Nottingham, about 60% of patients elect to call their general practitioner (GP) and they phone, on average, at just over 80 minutes after symptom onset. The GP arrives, makes a diagnosis and, if necessary, calls an ambulance. The ambulance journey time to hospital is between ten and twenty minutes. Then there is the inevitable delay in hospital before transfer to the coronary care unit.

In comparison, patients who elect to call emergency 999 still delay before the telephone call, on average over 60 minutes, but they arrive in hospital some two and a half times quicker than patients who elect for a first call to their GP (Fig. 1).

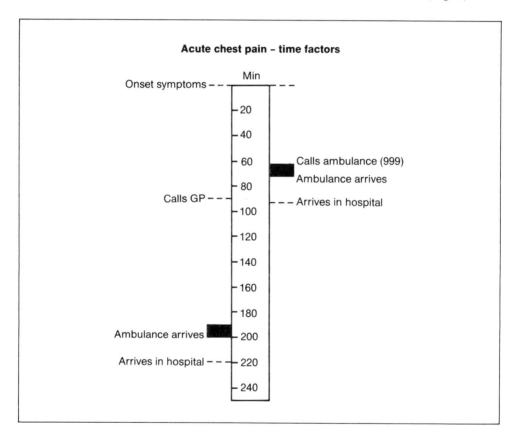

Fig. 1. Time ladder. Typical response times from onset of symptoms to arrival in hospital according to GP or 999 call.

Many behavioural questions may be asked to investigate the patient and GP response. Two merit particular attention: "Can we get patients to call earlier?" and "What do GPs think is their role in this new era of urgent thrombolytic treatment?".

Encouraging early calls for help

This problem was addressed at the Department of Medicine, University Hospital, Nottingham, a few years ago — when around 15,000 adults above the age of 40 years belonging to four participating general practices were sent a non-alarming letter explaining the potential significance of acute chest pain and inviting them to ring a 'heart watch' number as an alternative to their GP [5]. Stickers bearing this number were provided for positioning around the recipient's home. The aim was to see whether this mailing had an effect on patients' behaviour in comparison with patients who were not similarly mailed.

A patient electing to call the heart watch number was immediately put through to the coronary care unit where a senior nurse would attempt to assess the urgency of the call. If the patient belonged to a heart watch practice and was at home, the dispatcher immediately sent the coronary car which carried a senior nurse from the coronary care unit and a senior house officer and all resuscitation equipment to the patient's home. If the patient was not in one of the study practices, or not at home, the dispatcher would arrange for the patient's GP to visit or would send an ambulance depending upon her assessment of the severity of the call.

Evaluating calls from the patients in the heart watch practices showed, firstly, there was a shortening of the time from onset of symptoms to phone call of about 40 minutes amongst those electing to phone the coronary care unit as opposed to those who called their GP, who then in turn immediately called the coronary care unit. Secondly, comparing the patients in the heart watch programme who elected to call their GPs with patients in non-heart watch practices or in the heart watch practices before the heart watch programme was set up, it can be seen that there was a shortening of the time between the onset of major symptoms and calling for help by the availability of this special telephone number (Fig. 2). About one-third of patients in the heart watch practices elected to call their GPs for various reasons (declared no knowledge of the scheme, worried about cost, not sure if symptoms relevant, preferred to speak to their GP, etc).

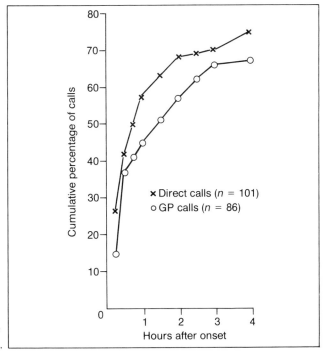

Fig. 2. Call times to GP compared with call times direct to special number in heartwatch practices after the mailing. More calls were made early to 411911 than to the GP.

The number of calls directly from the patients to the special number or to the GPs was different between patients with definite and probable myocardial infarction and those subsequently shown not to have infarcted. There were more telephone calls to the coronary care unit from patients without definite or probable infarctions than to the GPs (Fig. 3). Conversely, among those patients who had proven infarcts there was no such difference in calls (Fig. 4).

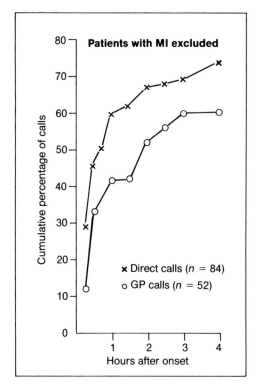

Fig. 3. Call times of patients *without* myocardial infarction at final diagnosis. More early calls to 411911 came from patients without definite or probable myocardial infarction.

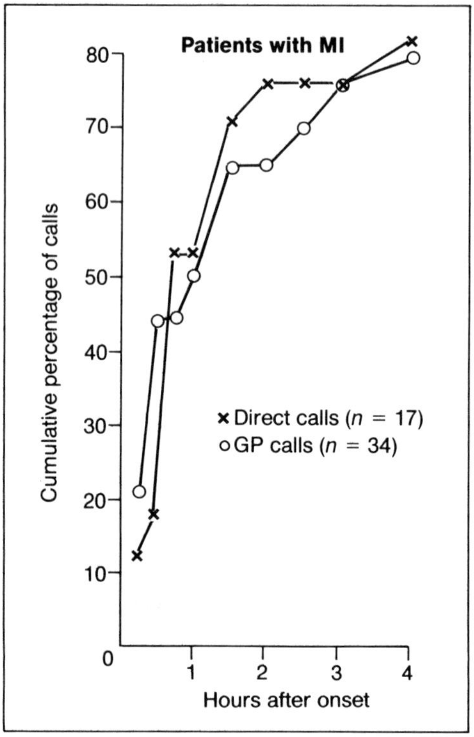

Fig. 4. Call times of patients *with* myocardial infarction at final diagnosis in heartwatch practices after the mailing. Calls to 411911 and to GPs were made equally early.

During this trial, it was interesting to note that the system was not flooded by a mass of patients calling about a lot of non-specific chest pain. In fact, about 60%-70% of the patients who either called the unit or their GPs eventually had a proven diagnosis of myocardial infarction. However, some patients were alarmed by the explanatory letter, indicating how sensitive an area patient education can be.

Role of the GP
The second question asked what involvement GPs would wish to have with their patients with acute chest pain out of hospital. During the winter of 1988/89, a postal survey was sent to some 600 general practitioners in South Nottinghamshire, asking whom a patient with acute chest pain should call in the first instance. The GPs were presented with three options: 1) the patient with a first episode of severe acute chest pain; 2) the patient with an episode of acute, severe chest pain who has already had a previous proven infarct; 3) the patient with acute, severe chest pain who already had

stable angina. About 20% of general practitioners thought that the patient, in all instances, should call the emergency 999 service (Fig. 5). About 5% thought the patients should take themselves immediately to the nearest casualty department, and about 75% would wish to be called by the patient in all circumstances.

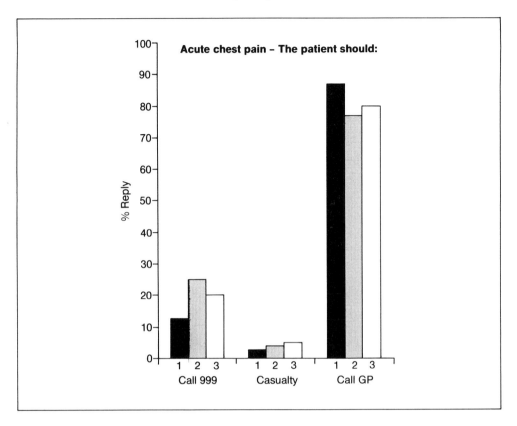

Fig. 5. What the patient should do. At onset of acute chest pain, the patient should... (1,2,3 — see text).

The GPs were then asked what they would advise if a patient called in the three instances above. About 80%-90% of the GPs said that they would visit the patient, and less than 10% would advise the patient to call 999 or go to casualty (Fig. 6). A few GPs would visit and also advise the patient to call 999. The majority of GPs who insisted on visiting the patient thought that they could do so within 30 minutes of the patient making the call. Epidemiological data suggest that this may be an optimistic estimate.

The GPs were also asked what sort of equipment they would carry if they were visiting patients with acute chest pain at home (Fig. 6). Very few of them have access to a defibrillator. One-fifth of the practices have an ECG although it is not always carried. The majority of GPs, however, carry some potentially useful cardiovascular drugs (morphine 96%, diuretic 96%, atropine 65%, lignocaine 32%).

On visiting the patient at home, some 70% of GPs would be prepared to keep at home some patients in whom they had made a diagnosis of acute myocardial infarction. There are various factors why they would elect to do so, such as social considerations, patient preference, and other severe life-limiting illnesses. Two factors had a strong influence. If the patient was much above the age of 65 years, many GPs

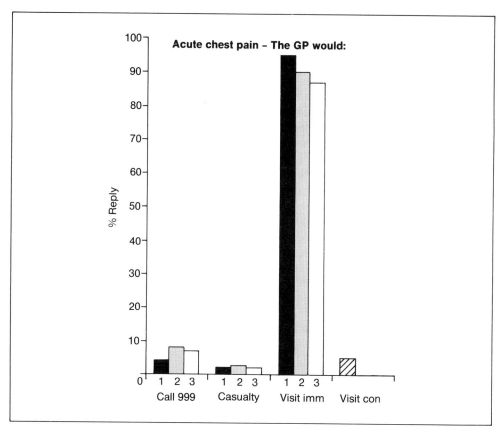

Fig. 6. What the GP would do. On receiving a call from a patient with acute chest pain, the GP would... (1,2,3 — see text; visit imm = visit immediately; visit con = visit when convenient).

(40%) would be prepared to keep that patient at home, even more (60%) if the patient was aged more than 75 years. If the patient had had symptoms for more than four to six hours, and provided there were no complications, 20% of GPs would be prepared to keep that patient at home, and over 50% if symptoms had begun more than 12 hours previously. It was estimated that about 15%-20% of patients in whom the GPs were making a diagnosis of myocardial infarction would, for various reasons, be kept at home. Interestingly, of those GPs who said they would always visit a patient with acute chest pain, one-quarter would never consider keeping patients at home and would always refer to hospital.

The GPs were also asked if, in this era of new treatments of thrombolysis, they would be prepared to institute thrombolytic therapy out of hospital. Sixty percent were prepared to do so provided the treatment could be given as a bolus, whereas only 14% were prepared to initiate out-of-hospital thrombolytic treatment if it were given by intravenous infusion. Many GPs made the point that they would be prepared to become involved in thrombolysis only after further instruction and further advice; for example, on whether ECG diagnosis is required and whether a defibrillator should be available in case arrhythmias occurred.

Conclusion

The survey in Nottingham indicates that the majority of GPs still wish to be involved in the management of out-of-hospital acute chest pain, and that many would be prepared to initiate thrombolytic therapy provided this could be given as a bolus injection. Many GPs lamented the loss of Nottingham's mobile coronary care system and would like to see it reinstated.

Patients are slow to accept changes in referral pattern but will do so and can be encouraged to call earlier, saving about 30-60 minutes. Earlier calls theoretically mean that patients would get into coronary care units within about one hour of onset of major symptoms (at present our mean delay is about three hours). Should patients therefore be encouraged to bypass the GP service or should they call both the GP and an ambulance? Should GPs and patients have access to a dedicated telephone, as Hillis and Dunn have introduced in Glasgow [6]?

GPs and their local cardiovascular physicians should, with the help of the ambulance service, agree upon a policy of rapid response to a patient with chest pain, especially if time is considered of prime importance for thrombolytic therapy.

References

[1] GISSI.
Effect of intravenous treatment in acute myocardial infarction.
Lancet 1986; **i:** 397–402.

[2] AIMS Trial Study Group.
Effect of intravenous APSAC on mortality after acute myocardial infarction: preliminary report of a placebo-controlled clinical trial.
Lancet 1988; **i:** 545–9.

[3] ISIS-2 (Second International Study of Infarct Survival) Collaborative Group.
Randomised trial of intravenous streptokinase, oral aspirin, both, or neither among 17187 cases of suspected acute myocardial infarction. ISIS-2.
Lancet 1988; **ii:** 349–60.

[4] ASSET Study Group.
Trial of tissue plasminogen activator for mortality reduction in acute myocardial infarction. Anglo-Scandinavian Study of Early Thrombolysis (ASSET).
Lancet 1988; **ii:** 525–30.

[5] Rowley JM, Hill JD, Hampton JR, Mitchell JRA.
Early reporting of myocardial infarction: impact of an experiment in patient education.
Br Med J 1982; **284:** 1741–6.

[6] Burns JMA, Hogg KJ, Rae AP, Hillis WS, Dunn FG.
Impact of a policy of direct admission to a coronary care unit on use of thrombolytic treatment.
Br Heart J 1989; **61:** 322–5.

RECENT CONCEPTS IN THE PREVENTION OF VENTRICULAR FIBRILLATION

R.W.F. CAMPBELL

The heart is a relatively simple organ with few specialized cells. It has a limited number of failure modes. Ventricular fibrillation (VF) is probably the most frequent and may, in electrophysiological terms, be regarded as the final common failure mode for a wide variety of cardiovascular disorders [1]. The cellular electrophysiology of VF itself will be similar in all these situations but it is the underlying pathophysiology that dictates prognosis and management.

This concept is illustrated by the three traces in Fig. 1. Trace A shows VF in a patient presenting with myocardial ischaemia but who has not suffered infarction. The immediate prognosis is good with the possibility of a near 100% restoration of sinus rhythm by direct current shock. Without further management however, the risk of recurrence is high. Such patients were first identified by out-of-hospital rescue squads, and initially the lack of underlying myocardial damage was interpreted as prognostically good. Follow-up revealed otherwise. The ischaemic circumstances creating the initial arrhythmia are not cured by resuscitation. Many patients have important underlying coronary artery disease on which may be superimposed repeated episodes of spasm or platelet aggregation, each bringing a risk of ischaemic VF.

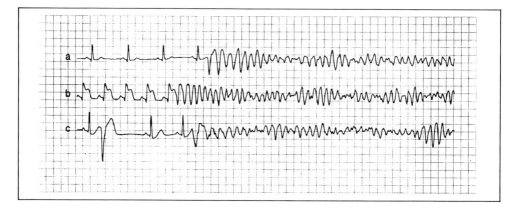

Fig. 1. Three incidents of ventricular fibrillation. A. Non-infarct ischaemic VF. B. Primary VF complicating acute myocardial infarction. C. Secondary ventricular fibrillation complicating acute myocardial infarction.

Trace B is from a patient who developed VF four hours after the onset of a myocardial infarction. He had neither shock nor cardiac failure. Restoration of sinus rhythm can be achieved in approximately 93% of such patients. The subsequent prognosis is good and after 12 hours, the recurrence rate is very low. The pathophysiology of this type of VF depends upon the transient unstable electrical conditions in ischaemic and actively infarcting myocardium. As the cells die, electrical stability is restored. Such primary VF (myocardial infarction-related, without shock or failure) is largely unrelated to either the size or site of infarction.

In trace C, VF occurs in a patient who has sustained a myocardial infarction and who is in shock and heart failure (secondary VF). Despite the cellular electrophysiology being nearly identical to that of patient B, the success rate for restoration of sinus rhythm is at best little more than 50% with a subsequent high hospital mortality for those resuscitated. Only 20% of those with secondary VF can be expected to leave hospital. The subsequent prognosis classically has been considered poor, but recent analysis of a study at Freeman Hospital suggests otherwise.

These examples demonstrate that it is the arrhythmogenic pathophysiology rather than the resultant electrophysiology which perhaps should command our attention in the management of VF.

Prognosis of VF
The prognosis of VF as it affects acute myocardial infarction has been the subject of

many reports since the earliest days of coronary care. Most have concentrated on the fate of hospital survivors. In a study of over 150 incidents of VF from my own hospital, the results of initial resuscitation, the hospital course and discharge follow-up (up to five years) have been investigated. Heart failure status emerged as the most important variable for initial resuscitation success and for survival of the hospital phase.

Site of infarction has been suggested as having a major impact on post-hospital prognosis. Schwartz *et al.* [2] reported a 32% one year mortality in patients surviving VF complicating an anterior infarction. The comparable figure for inferior infarcts was 6%. We have been unable to confirm this site-specific effect on prognosis.

VF types in acute myocardial infarction
Three types of VF have been discussed — non-infarct ischaemic VF, primary VF complicating acute myocardial infarction and secondary VF complicating acute infarction. Subtypes of VF can also be distinguished with respect to the underlying pathophysiological process taking place during the infarct process: acute occlusional VF, acute phase post-occlusional VF, reperfusional VF and late phase VF.

Acute occlusional VF
This type of VF occurs in the first few minutes of coronary artery occlusion and is responsible for the majority of sudden cardiac deaths occurring outside hospital. Formal investigation of this type of VF is extremely difficult but there is circumstantial evidence suggesting that beta-adrenoreceptor blocking drugs may sometimes prevent its occurrence.

Acute phase post-occlusional VF
This VF (indistinguishable electrocardiographically from the other types of VF) occurs within the first 12 hours of acute myocardial infarction. It is the VF seen mostly in coronary care units. Prophylactic lignocaine, beta-adrenoreceptor blocking drugs and magnesium reduce its incidence.

Reperfusional VF
This form of VF is unusual in man perhaps because, as yet, lytically induced reperfusion occurs relatively late after coronary artery occlusion. Animal experiments initially had raised fears that reperfusional VF would limit the practical use of thrombolytic therapy. Spontaneous thrombolysis occurs in human infarction but usually late and it is unlikely to contribute to VF occurring in coronary care units. Lignocaine has been shown to be ineffective for the prophylaxis of reperfusional VF [3]. At present, this arrhythmic complication is best treated when it arises. Reperfusional VF may signify a good prognosis as its occurrence probably requires the electrical reactivation of a substantial mass of myocardium.

Late phase VF
Late phase VF occurs more than 24 hours after the acute occlusion. Some incidents may reflect new ischaemia but others are related to the extent of underlying myocardial damage and may arise through degeneration of haemodynamically significant ventricular tachycardia. The beneficial effects on mortality seen in post-infarct survivors treated with beta-adrenoreceptor blocking drugs may be due to protection from this type of VF.

VF prevention in coronary care units
Currently there is no ideal management strategy against the risk of VF in infarct

patients admitted to a coronary care unit. Ample evidence exists that such VF cannot be predicted on the basis of monitoring for prior 'warning arrhythmias' [4]. VF is time dependent, however, such that its risk declines exponentially as the infarct matures. The association of VF and hypokalaemia is neither sensitive nor specific. In a study in Newcastle-upon-Tyne, the risk of VF was 8% in patients with admission potassiums of <3 mmol/l and 0.9% in patients with potassium levels >4 mmol/l. Of the 25 patients with low potassiums (<3mmol/l) only two developed VF, the others had an uncomplicated course [5].

Three studies have confirmed that prophylactic lignocaine can reduce the risk of VF, but in the latest and most comprehensive investigation [6] the VF reduction was associated with a significant risk of asystole, raising serious doubts about the cost-utility of such prophylaxis. Beta-adrenoreceptor blocking drugs and magnesium may have a role in preventing VF but despite encouraging reports, their use in the United Kingdom has not become routine.

If general prophylaxis is not used and VF is not predictable, then the only remaining management strategy is to await the occurrence of VF and to treat it promptly. Such is now the most common approach in British Coronary Care Units. Unfortunately not all patients even with primary VF can be resuscitated to sinus rhythm, raising concern that perhaps the search for effective prophylaxis should continue. There is no evidence however, that those who die of primary VF would have been salvageable; some may have suffered their VF as a consequence of a further and non-survivable coronary artery occlusion.

Predicting and preventing late VF
Secondary prevention of infarct survivors has been well researched. The high risk survivors of myocardial infarction can be identified by a variety of features although few if any of these reflect a direct propensity to VF. Rather they relate to the extent and severity of the underlying disease and the index infarction. Thus continuing angina, a poor effort tolerance, cardiomegaly and heart failure identify the high risk patients, but their demise may not necessarily be arrhythmic.

Much interest has centred on the prognostic significance of ventricular ectopic beats post-infarction. At rates of >10 per hour they carry independent prognostic significance. It has been tempting to extrapolate from ectopic beats to ventricular tachycardia and VF as the mechanism of death but this relationship is not substantiated. Antiarrhythmic drug trials to reduce ventricular ectopic beats with the hope of improving prognosis have failed, most spectacularly with the Cardiac Arrhythmia Suppression Trial (CAST) in which a significant excess mortality occurred in patients randomized to receive the Class Ic agents encainide and flecainide [7]. Beta-adrenoreceptor blocking drugs do offer mortality improvements and although disputed, may do so through an anti-VF effect.

The advent of signal averaging to define late activation of ventricular myocardium post-infarction has allowed the identification of infarct survivors at risk of sustained ventricular tachycardia and sudden death. The feature is one of a few which may directly identify an arrhythmogenic substrate. Patients with signal averaged late potentials probably are best managed by invasive, electrophysiologically guided antiarrhythmic therapy.

VF management — the real problem
It is taking a surprisingly long time to understand the mechanisms which underlie VF in man. The basic anatomic, biochemical and physiological processes in infarction

provide a framework for the electrophysiological disturbances, but in individual patients the particular mechanism for their VF is difficult or impossible to establish. Moreover, as VF depends upon many factors, some of which may arise only seconds before the arrhythmia starts, reliable prediction of these events is unlikely. Most episodes of VF occur out-of-hospital. Paramedic rescue squads are beginning to have some impact on the problem but it is clear from the North American experience that successful out-of-hospital VF management depends in part upon a high level of cardiopulmonary resuscitation skills being present in the community. The human heart can tolerate VF for long periods of time but the lack of cardiac output causes irreversible damage in other vital organs. With only four minutes to spare between the onset of VF and changes that lead inexorably to cerebral death, resuscitation must be swift and efficient.

References

[1] Campbell RWF.
Ventricular fibrillation — facts, fiction and the future. In: Hearse DJ, Manning AS, Janse MJ, eds. *Life threatening arrhythmias during ischaemia and infarction.*
New York: Raven Press, 1987; 1–9.

[2] Schwartz PJ, Zaza A, Grazi S, *et al.*
Effects of ventricular fibrillation complicating acute myocardial infarction on long term prognosis. Influence of site of infarction.
Am J Cardiol 1985; **57:** 384–9.

[3] Kertes P, Hunt D.
Prophylaxis of primary ventricular fibrillation in acute myocardial infarction. The case against lignocaine.
Br Heart J 1984; **52:** 241–7.

[4] Campbell RWF, Murray A, Julian DG.
Ventricular arrhythmias in first 12 hours of acute myocardial infarction. Natural history study.
Br Heart J 1981; **46:** 351–7.

[5] Campbell RWF, Higham D, Adams P, Murray A.
Potassium — its relevance for arrhythmias complicating acute myocardial infarction.
J Cardiovasc Pharm 1987; **10:** S25–7.

[6] Koster RW, Dunning AJ.
Intramuscular lidocaine for prevention of lethal arrhythmias in the prehospitalisation phase of acute myocardial infarction.
N Engl J Med 1985; **313:** 1105–10.

[7] The Cardiac Arrhythmia Suppression Trial (CAST) Investigators.
Preliminary report: effect of encainide and flecainide on mortality in a randomised trial of arrhythmia suppression after myocardial infarction.
N Engl J Med 1989; **321:** 406–12.

THE FUTURE OF THE CARDIAC CARE UNIT. CAN WE MAKE IT MORE EFFECTIVE?

S.M. COBBE

Introduction

Improving the therapy offered by coronary care units (CCUs) has been a central theme of this meeting. However, it is also important to look at the organization of the CCU to identify any improvements that may be made. Such a review entails scrutiny of the whole sequence of admission, assessment, treatment and discharge. Even on a superficial viewing, patient delay, delay by the general practitioner (GP), ambulance delay, procedures in the accident and emergency department, the operating practice of the CCU itself and the discharge policy may be identified as just some of the areas where increased organizational efficiency may yield dividends in terms of patient wellbeing. Critical audit of this field demands the collection of prospective data, and a review of the prospective information presently available is a natural starting point for discussion.

Delay to admission at the CCU

Table 1 shows data from a coronary care project in the Aberdeen area of Scotland [1]. A group of highly motivated, well equipped GPs gave absolute priority to emergency calls from patients with suspected acute myocardial infarction. Median patient delay was two hours, with an unusually high proportion of patients (66%) seeking help within four hours of the onset of symptoms. Median doctor delay was 15 minutes. These times are quite exceptional and probably cannot be matched anywhere else in the UK, unless comparable groups of enthusiasts emerge.

Table 1. Patient and general practioner delays in acute myocardial infarction. (After Rawles JM, Haites NE. *Br Med J* 1988; 296: 882–5. [1])

Patient and GP delays in acute MI
450 patients seen by GPs
Median patient delay 2 h
Median doctor delay 15 min
Two-thirds of patients sought help within 4 h

Some interesting observations were made in this study. Patient delay, for instance, correlated with age. This is reassuring in that treatment can be concentrated on the younger patient with acute myocardial infarction although, of course, the data suggest that thrombolytic therapy is worthwhile in the older patient as well [2]. Another interesting observation was that doctor delay correlated with patient delay, indicating that the degree of urgency which the patient transmitted to the doctor influenced the doctor's response. Doctor delay was also related to the ultimate place of treatment, suggesting that if the doctor had already decided that the patient would be managed at home, he did not attend quite so quickly.

Coronary care admission policies can be altered by streamlining the procedure in the case of patients who have been seen by their GP. Data from Stewart Hillis' unit at Stobhill General Hospital, Glasgow, illustrate this (Fig. 1) [3]. Stobhill Hospital is on the outskirts of the city; it is possible to bring an ambulance to the back door of the CCU where there is a small assessment room. For patients assessed by their GP and sent directly to the CCU the mean delay from onset of symptoms to admission was substantially shorter than in those processed through the accident and emergency department, despite the fact that the delay from onset of symptoms to the patient's call for help was not significantly different. This difference in being seen by a GP translated into clear clinical benefits, in that the percentage of patients admitted within three hours of the onset of pain was improved and the percentage receiving thrombolytic therapy was increased. At the time of this study a rather restricted policy was in force, limiting thrombolysis to people seen within four hours. Clearly then, where it is possible, there can be advantages in arranging an assessment by a GP and direct admission to the CCU.

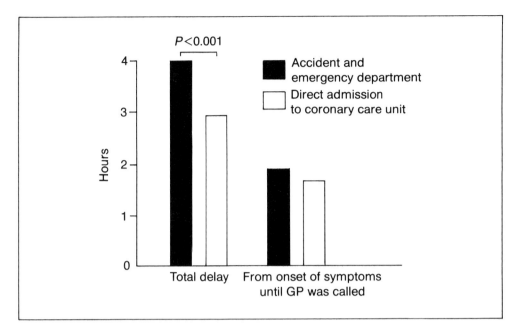

Fig. 1. Delay from onset of symptoms to admission and treatment was reduced in patients assessed by their GPs and sent directly to the coronary care unit. (Reproduced with permission from Burns JMA, Hogg KJ, Rae AP, Hillis WS, Dunn FG. *Br Heart J* 1989; **61**: 322–5. [3])

Recent experience at the neighbouring Glasgow Royal Infirmary is worth looking at. This is a city centre hospital at which ambulance access to the CCU is restricted. A survey in 1985 revealed that 65% of admissions with chest pain were the result of self-referrals. Of these patients presenting to the casualty department, 44% were judged to have chest pain of cardiac origin. The largest single cause of self-referral for chest pain was alcoholic gastritis. Over the past year a prospective audit has been conducted to determine the strengths and weaknesses of the existing system for processing and treating patients. During the audit period, 817 admissions to CCU were recorded, 246 (30%) of which were initially diagnosed as acute myocardial infarction. The policy with regard to the administration of streptokinase was to treat patients admitted within six hours of the onset of symptoms provided that ST segment elevation was evident on the ECG. Applying this criterion, 131 patients (53%) received thrombolytic therapy. Ninety-one patients did not receive thrombolytic therapy because of a time delay >6 hours since the onset of symptoms, or because of insufficient ECG evidence of infarction. Another 24 patients admitted with suspected acute myocardial infarction had contraindications to the use of thrombolytic therapy. In only five cases overall was failure to administer streptokinase attributable to delays in the casualty department.

These five cases represent a disappointing failure and show that there is room for improvement, but overall the picture is moderately encouraging. An overview of the efficiency of the system is obtained from a consideration of the time between onset of symptoms and start of thrombolytic therapy. This commendably simple measure will reflect all the delays encountered in the system. In this case, streptokinase was administered to 50% of the 131 patients within two and a half hours.

One interesting point to emerge from the study was the impact of feedback on response times. Following review of performance in the first six month period, response-time curves were shifted to the left during the next period of six months, suggesting such reviews may be a useful aid to staff motivation.

One final finding to emerge from this study was that patients selected for streptokinase therapy tended to be processed faster from casualty to CCU than people who were not. While this is understandable, it would be preferrable that those not selected for streptokinase therapy should also reach the CCU more rapidly, since facilities for defibrillation are better there.

Selection of patients for treatment

The issue of selecting patients for management in a CCU requires attention. In 1984 Pozen conducted a study among 2800 patients using a programme in a hand-held calculator to predict the likelihood of ensuing acute myocardial infarction in patients assessed in the casualty department [4]. This technique resulted in a reduction in the number of patients admitted to the CCU who turn out not to have acute infarction. Equally important, there was no increase in the number of people inappropriately discharged home from the casualty department. Such findings may have major financial implications — admission to a CCU is costly and false admissions represent an often avoidable drain on scarce resources.

Costs of treatment

The cost entailed in admission is outlined in Table 2, which draws on US estimates to compare the costs of four alternative treatment options [5]. In this classification, 'routine' means care on a general medical ward. Most UK CCUs would come under the heading of 'intermediate CCUs', the category 'CCU' being reserved for the more lavishly equipped units in the USA. Just to admit the patient to hospital costs US$ 283,000 per life year saved (1980 prices). The further (incremental) cost of admission to an intermediate unit that offers monitoring and defibrillation facilities is relatively small, whereas admission to a unit meeting the US definition of a CCU imposes enormous incremental costs.

Table 2. Cost-effectiveness of coronary care unit admission versus intermediate care according to probability of myocardial infarction. (After Fineberg HV, Scadden D, Goldman L. N Engl J Med 1984; 310: 1301–7. [5])

	Dollars (1980)	
Probability %	Costs per life × 10^6	Costs per life year
5	2.04	139,000
10	0.97	66,000
20	0.49	33,000

The conclusion from this cost analysis is that if a patient is going to be admitted to hospital then the best value is offered by an intermediate care unit. Use should be made of a greater number of monitored beds with less intense nursing supervision.

Step-down units or telemetered beds are the obvious way in which this could be achieved at relatively acceptable cost. The other important message from this study relates to the previous study by Pozen in terms of diagnostic accuracy. The authors calculated the cost-effectiveness of (US-style) CCU versus intermediate care according to the probability that the patient had myocardial infarction. Not surprisingly, as the probability that the person had myocardial infarction increased, the cost per life year saved decreased. In other words, the more carefully and successfully patients are selected for admission to a highly expensive form of treatment, the better value for money that treatment is.

Early discharge from the CCU

Another element in the cost equation is how quickly patients may be discharged from CCU. In the UK, the tendency is to keep patients in the CCU for 48 hours after infarction. They then go to a general medical ward and are discharged from hospital at about seven days. In 1988, Topol reviewed a policy of very aggressive early discharge in patients at day three, based on the patients having had an uncomplicated in-hospital course and a negative exercise thallium scan at the time of discharge [6]. The overall numbers eligible for early discharge according to this policy were not large, but they indicated that an early discharge policy may be more useful than most doctors realize. A total of 80 patients were randomized to discharge either at day three or, more conventionally, at days 7-10. The clinical outcome at six months was not different between the two groups; there were no deaths, no new ventricular aneurysms and similar rates of clinical recurrence. Overall, numbers returning to work in the two groups were the same. The delay before they returned to work was different, however. The group discharged early returned to work earlier, and this difference was greater than simply the added days patients discharged at days 7-10 spent in hospital. Importantly, the hospital cost in dollars was reduced from a mean of nearly US$ 18,000 to US$ 12,500 in patients discharged early. So clearly there is scope, in carefully selected patients, for much earlier hospital discharge than has previously been the case.

Conclusion

The effective use of CCU facilities entails a critical analysis of all aspects of the review of patients, admission to CCU, management within the unit and discharge. In the era of audit, data have to be collected on timings, performance, stay in hospital, stay in the CCU and, of course, outcome in order to make sure that resources are used optimally.

References

[1] Rawles JM, Haites NE.
Patient and general practitioner delays in acute myocardial infarction.
Br Med J 1988; **296:** 882–5.

[2] ISIS-2 (Second International Study of Infarct Survival Collaborative Group).
Randomized trial of intravenous streptokinase, oral aspirin, both or neither among 17187 cases of suspected acute myocardial infarction: ISIS-2.
Lancet 1988; **ii:** 249–50.

[3] Burns JMA, Hogg KJ, Rae AP, Hillis WS, Dunn FG.
Impact of a policy of direct admission to a coronary care unit on the use of thrombolytic treatment.
Br Heart J 1989; **61:** 322–5.

[4] Pozen MW, D'Agostin RB, Selker HP, Sytkowski PA, Hood WB Jr.
A predictive instrument to improve coronary-care-unit admission practices in acute ischaemic heart disease. A prospective multi-centre clinical trial.
N Engl J Med 1984; **310:** 1273–8.

[5] Fineberg HV, Scadden D, Goldman L.
     Care of patients with a low probability of
     acute myocardial infarction. Cost
     effectiveness of alternatives to coronary-care-
     unit admission.
     N Engl J Med 1984; **310**: 1301–7.

[6] Topol EJ, Burek K, O'Neill WW, *et al.*
     A randomized controlled trial of hospital
     discharge three days after myocardial
     infarction in the era of reperfusion.
     N Engl J Med 1988; **318**: 1083–8.

NEW OPPORTUNITIES IN PRE-HOSPITAL CARE

R. VINCENT

Introduction

Interest in pre-hospital care for patients with acute myocardial infarction (MI) arose from the challenge of early malignant arrhythmias [1]. This arrhythmic challenge remains, but is now accompanied by the new dimension of thrombolysis.

I should like to examine the provision of care for the infarct patient before hospital admission, reflecting on the various strategies on offer, and to review briefly the recent Brighton experience of treating patients who have sustained out-of-hospital ventricular fibrillation, usually as a result of acute ischaemia though not always of infarction.

The Cardiac Department at the Royal Sussex County Hospital in Brighton, which serves about 350,000 people, records 25-35 out-of-hospital rescues a year. While this achievement has no dramatic effect on overall mortality, it does establish that such salvage is feasible. In the aftermath of successful cardioversion, however, the further challenge of evolving myocardial necrosis often has to be confronted; a decision on strategies for continuing emergency medical care is unavoidable.

Equipment

New technologies have played a prominent part in extending the opportunities for pre-hospital care. For example, increasing use is being made — of automatic and semi-automatic defibrillators that can diagnose malignant ventricular arrhythmias and administer appropriate life-saving defibrillation with little or no operator intervention [2]. Comprehensive, on site electrocardiographic (ECG) evaluation can be valuable in the diagnosis of acute myocardial infarction before hospital admission [3]. Telephonic ECG monitoring, in practice, is more problematic; where a high level of skill in ECG monitoring already exists among ambulance crews or other emergency staff, it is probably redundant.

Newer mechanical aids to resuscitation range from external pacing [4] and defibrillation through devices for ventilation and airways support to more complex (and perhaps unnecessary) mechanical devices for chest compression.

Pharmacological intervention

The value of pain relief for patients with evolving myocardial infarction is widely agreed, not only for patient comfort but for the reduction of increased sympathetic tone, an important pre-disposing factor to ventricular arrhythmias. Opiates are established agents but there is a need for alternative drugs that can provide effective pain relief with less emetic action, less disturbance of blood pressure and, perhaps, less potential for the development of dependence.

In recent years pharmacological intervention to restore coronary flow has centred on thrombolysis [5-9]; but the value of vasodilators should not be ignored. Effort may profitably be spent on determining which forms of *nitrate* delivery system are most appropriate for use in pre-hospital care.

Finally, any prospect for an alternative to lignocaine as an antiarrhythmic for routine use that suppresses arrhythmias without resulting in bradycardia or myocardial depression would be welcome.

The role of the family doctor and the ambulance

Technical progress in recent years has added much to the quality of out-of-hospital care and further advance in this area may be anticipated. In parallel, however, attention must be focused closely on organizational aspects of pre-hospital treatment if it is to be used to full advantage.

The framework of pre-hospital care varies considerably from country to country, and it is impossible to define a simple, unified system. A feature common to most arrangements in the UK, however, is the triangular relationship between the hospital and the two main agencies of pre-hospital care, the family doctor and the ambulance service.

Family doctors have greater clinical skill and a more extensive knowledge of medicine than ambulance staff. But the average UK general practitioner (GP) sees relatively few cases of myocardial infarction in a year, so that his experience in ECG interpretation and management of such patients may be limited. In many instances, he may have access to only meagre facilities for monitoring and resuscitation.

The ambulance service is designed to offer a rapid response and in many places is likely to have better resuscitation facilities [10]. This will be particularly true in areas of Britain where extended training for ambulance crews is being adopted. As the National Health Service Training Authority programme of extended training gathers momentum, increasing numbers of ambulance staff trained in resuscitation and arrhythmia interpretation will be available for emergency care.

The final arm of this triad, the hospital, is, by definition, not part of pre-hospital care. Nevertheless, liaison of the hospital with the other two arms and its preparedness to invest in educational programmes is essential.

The ideal response to a patient with acute myocardial infarction would involve the complete triad: the near-simultaneous attendance of both the GP and the resuscitation ambulance crew in early radio contact with the admitting hospital.

Pre-hospital care in Brighton

Following the inception of a coronary ambulance service in the Brighton area, time to admission of patients with suspected acute myocardial infarction was shortened dramatically (Table 1). On first evaluation, this appears to be the direct result of improved response times on the part of the ambulances. Underlying this, however, is a more broadly-based change in the policy of admission in favour of early referral of patients with suspected myocardial infarction. Equally important was the effort put into informing GPs that the hospital welcomes early referrals.

Has the provision of a coronary ambulance service changed the pattern of referral for patients with myocardial infarction or suspected infarction? The answer would appear to be no (Table 2). Over the time that the service has been operating, the

Table 1.   Change in delay to hospital admission for patients with acute myocardial infarction as a result of the introduction of a Coronary Ambulance scheme in Brighton in 1972.

Delays to hospital admission

1971 : Median more than 6 h

1986 : Median approx. 2 h (Skilled care approx. 1 h 40 min)

Table 2.   Result of a community training programme in basic life support and the recognition of a coronary attack introduced in Brighton in 1982 on the pattern of referral of patients with acute myocardial infarction.

	1981	1988
Proportion patients first calling GP	42%	44%
Median time from onset of symptoms to ambulance call	1 h 26 min	1 h 56 min

proportion of patients bypassing their GP and summoning the ambulance directly has lain in the range 42%-45%. Thus, about half of the patients still contact their GP first, a figure not greatly at variance with that recorded in the days before the ambulance service was initiated. Since this well-publicised facility has been running for over 15 years,the public appears to have a very conservative response to innovation — or a resistance to publicity.

Public education has been another important strand in the Brighton policy for pre-hospital care [11]. Since 1978, some 40,000 people have been trained in the recognition of acute cardiac pain and in techniques for basic life support. Has this change in community knowledge affected the delay between onset of symptoms and the summoning of help? Again, the answer appears to be no. But despite this apparently disappointing finding, it would be wrong to discount community education programmes. Appreciable benefit from 'by-stander' intervention has been seen in many individual patients even if group statistics are unaffected by public education in cardiopulmonary resuscitation. There is no reason to abandon the premise that the more the public knows and understands, the better.

What are the prospects for the pre-hospital use of thrombolytic agents by paramedical staff? Discussions with staff of the Brighton ambulance service indicate that unexpected psychological barriers have to be dismantled before this prospect may be realized. Thrombolytic therapy is recognized as powerfully beneficial — but is also known to cause harm [12]. A major concern amongst ambulancemen relates to the issue of diagnosis. In the very early stages of infarction, ECG changes may be less than fully characteristic. Given that ambulance crews may be working in far from ideal circumstances, their apprehensions can be appreciated. In fact, such comparisons as we have made to-date indicate that ambulance crews are equally if not more reliable in their diagnosis than the junior doctors who examine patients on their arrival at hospital. But further extensive scrutiny of the performance of ambulance crews, supplemented where necessary by further training, will be needed to instill a greater sense of self-confidence in these staff responsible for patient care.

To help allay the crew's perception of thrombolysis as a treatment with capacity for harm [13], a screening protocol suitable for their use at the bedside has been drawn up (Fig. 1). Ambulance crews consider thrombolytic therapy only if affirmative answers are obtained to 18 separate questions. At present, crews are still engaged in a pilot study to confirm that their diagnostic acumen is sufficient to be applied without supervision; as yet they have given thrombolytic agents only in the presence of a doctor after the patient has arrived at hospital rather than in the field. Some while will elapse before unsupervised pre-hospital administration is sanctioned; more time still will be needed before the impact of such interventions can be judged.

THE AMBULANCE APSAC TRIAL

A. If you see a patient who may qualify for APSAC treatment, use any convient nearby telephone to call 688141. Say you require the Medical SHO urgently. If there is no convenient telephone ask control for channel 3 to contact A & E.

B. If you cannot establish contact with a doctor within 5 minutes then abort the attempt. We are trying to save time and we must not waste it.

PATIENT'S NAME: .... DATE: ....

AMBULANCEMEN WILL EXPECT TO ANSWER THE FOLLOWING QUESTIONS ABOUT ANY PATIENT CONSIDERED A CANDIDATE FOR PRE-HOSPITAL THROMBOLYTIC THERAPY.

TICK FOR YES

1. Can you confirm that the patient is not a woman of child-bearing age .... ☐
2. Is the patient aged 70 or less? .... ☐
3. Is the patient conscious and coherent? .... ☐
4. Has the patient had symptoms characteristic of a coronary heart attack (ie the pain in a typical distribution of 20 minutes duration or more)? .... ☐
5. Did the continuous symptoms start less than 6 hours ago? .... ☐
6. Does the electrocardiogram show ST segment elevation of 2mm or more (0.08 seconds after J point) in at least two standard leads or at least two precordial leads? .... ☐
7. Is the QRS width 0.12mm or less, and is bundle branch block absent from the tracing? ...... ☐
8. Can you confirm that there is NO atrioventricular block greater than 1st degree .... ☐
9. Did the pain build up over seconds and minutes rather than starting totally abruptly? .... ☐
10. Can you confirm that breathing does not influence the severity of the pain? .... ☐
11. Can you confirm that the patient has not been treated for a peptic ulcer within the last 12 months? .... ☐
12. Can you confirm that the patient has not had a stroke of any sort within the last 12 months? ... ☐
13. Can you confirm that the patient has no diagnosed bleeding tendency? .... ☐
14. Can you confirm that the patient has not had any surgical operation (including tooth extractions) within the last 4 weeks? .... ☐
15. Can you confirm definitely that APSAC/streptokinase has NOT been given within the last 6 months? .... ☐
16. Can you confirm that the heart rate is between 50 and 140? .... ☐
17. Can you confirm that the patient is not on warfarin? .... ☐
18. Can you confirm that the systolic BP is over 80mm? .... ☐

If the answer to all the above questions is YES, for the period of the trial the SHO will ask if the answer to all the questions is YES. You will reply "AFFIRMATIVE" and give an ETA for arrival in the A & E.

COMMENTS:- _____

_____ Signed: _____

NOTE: If patient has MI but does NOT qualify please send in form

Fig. 1. Screening protocol used by Extended Trained Ambulance personnel in the assessment for thrombolysis of a patient with suspected acute myocardial infarction.

Conclusion

New opportunities in pre-hospital care afforded by developments in technology, pharmacology, training and organization herald an exciting era of improved management of acute myocardial infarction. It remains for these opportunities to be made available on a wide scale.

References

[1] Briggs RS, Brown PM, Crabb ME, *et al.*
The Brighton resuscitation ambulances: a continuing experiment in pre-hospital care by ambulance staff.
Br Med J 1976; **2**: 1161–5.

[2] Cummins R, Eisenberg MS, Litwin PE, *et al.*
Automatic external defibrillators used by emergency medical technicians: a controlled clinical trial.
JAMA 1987; **257**: 1605–10.

[3] Gordon I.
Streptokinase used in general practice.
J R Coll Gen Pract 1989; **39**: 44–51.

[4] Hedges JR, Syverud SA, Dalsey WD.
Developments in transcutaneous and transthoracic pacing during bradysystolic arrest.
Ann Emerg Med 1984; **13**: 822–8.

[5] ISAM Study Group.
A prospective trial of intravenous streptokinase in acute myocardial infarction (ISAM). Mortality, morbidity and infarct size at 21 days.
N Engl J Med 1986; **314**: 1465–71.

[6] GISSI.
Effectiveness of intravenous thrombolytic treatment in acute myocardial infarction.
Lancet 1986; **i**: 397–402.

[7] ISIS-2 (Second International Study of Infarct Survival) Collaborative Group.
Randomised trial of intravenous streptokinase, oral aspirin, both or neither among 17,187 cases of suspected myocardial infarction: ISIS-2.
Lancet 1988; **ii**: 349–60.

[8] AIMS Trial Study Group.
Effect of intravenous APSAC on mortality after acute myocardial infarction: preliminary report of a placebo-controlled clinical trial.
Lancet 1988; **i**: 545–9.

[9] Wilcox RG, von der Lippe G, Olsson CG, Jenson G, Skene AM, Hampton JR.
Trial of tissue plasminogen activator for mortality reduction in acute myocardial infarction: Anglo-Scandinavian study of early thrombolysis (ASSET).
Lancet 1988; **ii**: 525–30.

[10] Vincent R.
Resuscitation by ambulance crews. In: Evans TR, ed. ABC of Resuscitation.
Br Med J 1986; **293**: 19–21.

[11] Vincent R, Martin B, Williams G, *et al.*
A community training scheme in cardiopulmonary resuscitation.
Br Med J 1984; **288**: 617–20.

[12] Erlemeir H-H, Zangemeister W, Burmester L, *et al.*
Bleeding after thrombolysis in acute myocardial infarction.
Eur Heart J 1989; **10**: 16–23.

[13] Yusuf S, Collins R, Peto R, *et al.*
Intravenous and intracoronary fibrinolytic therapy in acute myocardial infarction: overview of results on mortality, reinfarction and side-effects from 33 randomised controlled trials.
Eur Heart J 1985; **6**: 556–85.

THE COST OF NEW THERAPIES

M.J. BUXTON

As medical science advances, and the possible ways of benefitting patients multiply, it becomes self-evident that choices have to be made as to how best to use the resources available to health services. Thus, the subjects of costs, of cost-effectiveness, and of economic analysis appear more and more prominently in the pages of clinical journals and in the proceedings of clinical medical conferences.

Concepts of economic evaluation

There is still, however, misunderstanding about economic evaluation in health care, and confusion persists over the economic terminology. The first point to emphasize is that economics is concerned with costs and benefits. Indeed, costs are simply a measure of the value forgone elsewhere in using resources in a particular way. Hence when economists talk of the benefits of health care interventions, they refer to the improvements in the health of patients (in terms of length or quality of life). Cost savings are not benefits. If that were the case, the way to achieve the greatest benefit from any health care system would be to close it down, so achieving maximum savings!

Economic evaluation can take a number of forms: four main categories are now fairly consistently distinguished in the literature from the UK, Europe and North America. Each of them measures costs in essentially the same way, but each handles health benefits differently. These four approaches are summarized in Table 1.

Cost-minimization analysis ignores the benefits, looks simply at costs, and establishes the least-cost alternative. This simple approach is very powerful, if the clinical equivalence of the alternatives has been well-demonstrated, or where there is no evidence as to differences in benefits. Additionally, it can be used where one alternative is indisputably superior in all dimensions of benefit, and where cost-minimization analysis can show that the better alternative is also the cheaper. Unfortunately, the better alternative is frequently more expensive, and in such circumstances one of the other three techniques must be employed to see whether the extra benefits are sufficient to justify the extra costs.

Cost-effectiveness analysis is the most common form of economic analysis. It takes a single measure of benefit that is most appropriate to the main objective of the intervention — for example, cholesterol level or life-years saved — and compares how much benefit can be achieved at what cost. This is particularly useful in comparing very similar alternatives.

However, interventions frequently have effects on more than one dimension of health benefit. *Cost-utility analysis* attempts to measure the relative value of different combinations of health characteristics. The most common expression of this multi-dimensional measure of benefit is the QALY (quality-adjusted life-year), which incorporates measures of length and quality of life. It is potentially a very powerful tool for comparing uses of resources in the health service, which offer quite different benefits to different patient groups.

Although the term is often used loosely, true *cost-benefit analysis*, the fourth category of economic evaluation, is problematic and few examples exist in the health-care literature. It measures all benefits in monetary terms, so assigning monetary values to health benefits such as life-years gained, or handicap prevented. Not surprisingly, the problem is to find acceptable methods for eliciting such monetary values, particularly the value for life itself.

Measuring costs

The common element in each of these approaches is a measurement of costs. From where should these estimates be obtained? What level of detail is required? Do costs estimates have to be based on actual observation, or can they be hypothetical? It is certainly true that frequently, in papers taken from good clinical trials, conclusions are

Table 1. Major forms of economic analysis. (Adapted from Drummond MF, *et al.* [1])

Type of analysis	Measurement/ valuation of costs in both alternatives	Capability for handling of 'health benefits' (positive or negative)	Measurement/ valuation of 'health benefits'
Cost-minimization analysis	Monetary	Only if identical in all relevant respects	None within analysis
Cost-effectiveness analysis	Monetary	Single effect of interest, common to both alternatives, but achieved to different degrees	Natural units (e.g. life-years gained, cure rate, points of blood pressure reduction, etc)
Cost-utility analysis	Monetary	Single or multiple effects, not necessarily common to both alternatives, and common effects may be achieved to different degrees by the alternatives	Effects encapsulated in single index most usually quality-adjusted life-years
Cost-benefit analysis	Monetary	Single or multiple effects, not necessarily common to both alternatives, and common effects may be achieved to different degrees by the alternatives	Monetary

drawn about costs based on very weak, hypothetical estimates. In some cases this may be quite sufficient, but the potential limitations must be recognized.

Indeed, trials themselves restrict the scope for differences in costs between the two arms, in that the protocol constrains the clinicians' ability to manage patients differentially. If the trial design requires that all patients undergo a battery of tests on day 10 after the intervention, patients are unlikely to be discharged on day eight even though that might be good clinical management for some: thus a potentially valuable difference in resource implications might not emerge from trial data.

It is also important to think about the cost period. It is generally easy to identify differences in the initial treatment period or the hospital stay, but important cost differences may exist in the longer term. What are the costs per case over a period of, for example, six months or a year? Are patients re-admitted more frequently or do they require more out-patient care with particular regimens?

When considering costs, it is important to consider who will be bearing the costs and from whose perspective they need to be analysed: the patient, the clinician's budget, the clinical specialty, the hospital, the health service, the public sector, or society as a whole. It is important not to confuse low cost interventions with high cost interventions that simply transfer costs away from a particular budget in question.

Example 1: Early discharge

A recent study by Topol *et al.* [2], already referred to by Stuart Cobbe (page 143), randomly assigned uncomplicated patients after myocardial infarction to early (day 3) discharge or conventional (days 7-10) discharge. With very full data on hospital and professional fees over a six-month period of follow-up, they came to the not unexpected conclusion that there was a statistically high significant difference in costs between these two groups ($12,546 compared to $17,868: $P<0.0001$). The trial evidence pointed to equal efficacy and equal benefit. However, doubts about the possible clinical differences led the authors to the cautious conclusion that "before this strategy can be widely recommended, however, its safety must be confirmed in larger prospective clinical trials." Arguably, because of the firm evidence of costs advantages, and the absence of evidence of disbenefit to the patient, early discharge should be recommended until any evidence arises to question its equal efficacy.

Avoiding unnecessary prolongation of stay provides a very easy opportunity to reduce costs, but frequently it is implied that existing patterns of discharge result from careful consideration of what is best for each case. Recently, we undertook in the Health Economics Research Group at Brunel University an analysis of data from a survey of physicians, in which they provided data on recent cases of acute myocardial infarction. The distribution of lengths of stay (Fig. 1) clearly shows peaks at days 8, 10, 14 and 21, reflecting standard policies or fixed organisational arrangements rather than a natural curve reflecting decisions on the most appropriate length of stay for specific patients.

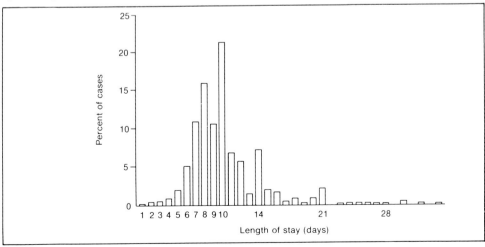

Fig. 1.   Length of inpatient stay for acute myocardial infarction (n = 649 UK case histories).

155

Example 2: Thrombolysis

The published literature now includes a number of good cost-effectiveness studies. For example, Vermeer *et al.* [3] present very useful data from a randomized trial in the Netherlands of early thrombolytic treatment with intracoronary streptokinase. They present data on mean life expectancy (estimated on the basis of reperfusion rates) and cost, and thus cost per life-year gained. As shown in Table 2, their results indicate the very much higher costs per life-year from inferior infarctions and from admissions more than two hours after onset.

This variability of cost-effectiveness is demonstrated even more clearly in a study by Laffel, Fineberg & Braunwald [4] that models the costs and survival benefits of a number of thrombolysis/reperfusion strategies. It shows the enormous range in costs per additional survivor from the use of t-PA, according to infarct size and rapidity of administration. The cost per additional survivor if used after more than four hours on a small infarct is more than fifty times greater than when used in under two hours on a large infarct (Table 3). This implies that a strictly selective policy for the use of thrombolysis will be much more cost-effective than blanket use. But are clinicians prepared to use such a policy to draw the dividing line between those who receive thrombolysis and those who do not?

Table 2. Calculation of costs (Dfl) per year of life gained in various groups of patients. (After Vermeer, *et al.* [3])

	Mean life expectancy (yr)		Costs		Costs per year of life gained
	C	T	C	T	
All patients	15.3	16.8	21 000	29 000	5 300
Inferior infarction	16.3	17.0	21 000	28 000	10 000
Anterior infarction (all patients)	14.1	16.5	20 000	29 000	3 800
Anterior infarction (admission $\leqslant$ 2 h and Σ ST $\geqslant$ 1.2 mV)	12.7	16.3	18 000	25 000	1 900
Anterior infarction (admission 2-4 h or Σ ST $<$ 1.2 mV)	15.1	16.6	22 000	32 000	6 700

Table 3. Incremental costs of t-PA (relative to conventional management): cost (thousand $ US) per additional survivor. (Adapted from Laffel, *et al.* [4])

	Infarct size		
Hours after infarct	Large	Moderate	Small
0	11	42	132
2	15	65	224
4	30	158	631

Example 3: Implantable defibrillators

Interpreting the implications of cost-effectiveness data can be difficult, particularly where the only available data reflects patient management in other countries. For example, from the USA Kupperman et al. [5] estimate that the use of the implantable defibrillator increases life expectancy for appropriate patients from approximately 3.2 to 5.1 years at an additional cost of $33,000, giving an estimated cost per life-year saved of approximately $18,000. We are currently undertaking some analysis of what the position might be in the UK context. Even if the costs relating to defibrillator patients are similar, the costs and effectiveness of current therapy may be very different. It seems likely that in the UK, cheaper but less effective empiric drug therapy is much more common than in the US where intensive electrophysiological testing is the norm. Thus it is possible that in the UK the increases in costs and in benefits from the use of the implantable defibrillator would both be greater than in the US.

Conclusions

The current interest in cost-effectiveness is slowly being matched by a growing number of good economic studies in the health service literature. These need to be used cautiously and interpreted with care, with due acknowledgement of the specific comparisons they make, and of the specific health care system context in which they are made. As with clinical studies, precise results may not be generalisable, and details may have to be questioned. All studies need a firm underpinning of sound clinical evidence. But increasingly such studies can begin to help clinicians question whether new therapies, or indeed old ones, represent the most effective use of the scarce health-care resources they command.

References

[1] Drummond MF, Stoddard GL, Torrance GW.
Methods for the economic evaluation of health care programmes.
Oxford: Oxford Medical Publications, 1987.

[2] Topol EJ, Burek K, O'Neill WW, et al.
A randomized controlled trial of hospital discharge three days after myocardial infarction in the era of reperfusion.
N Engl J Med 1988; **318:** 1083–8.

[3] Vermeer F, Simoons ML, de Zwaan C, et al.
Cost benefit analysis of early thrombolytic treatment with intracoronary streptokinase.
Br Heart J 1988; **59:** 527–34.

[4] Laffel GL, Fineberg HV, Braunwald E.
A cost-effectiveness model for coronary thrombolysis/reperfusion therapy.
J Am Coll Cardiol 1987; **10:** 79B–90B.

[5] Kupperman M, Luce BR, McGovern B, et al.
An analysis of the cost effectiveness of the implantable defibrillator.
Circulation 1990; **81:** 91–100.

MAKING THE MOST OF THE CARDIAC CARE BUDGET

D. CHAMBERLAIN

Introduction

In the United Kingdom, we have had intensive care for cardiac patients for around thirty years and the concept of pre-hospital care was developed nearly twenty-five years ago. Yet despite this head start over the rest of the world, the twins of coronary care and pre-hospital care have not prospered in the United Kingdom. They were weakened, maybe, by the diseases of doubt and, above all, by complacency. Furthermore, the care of coronary patients in Britain has not been in the hands of cardiologists but, mostly, in the hands of general physicians. The situation is now improving, with more cardiologists, physicians who are better educated, the development of new exciting therapeutic possibilities, a better informed medical profession in general and, to a degree, better informed patients. Problems still exist, of course, one of which is increasingly stringent cost constraints. Ways have to be found of taking advantage of the new opportunities but they must be both sensible and economical to make the most of the cardiac care budget.

Treatment is expensive and undeniably now highly effective; but in relative terms it is not important which drugs are used. The logistics and the salaries needed to provide high technology medicine represent the greatest costs. It is probably fair to say too that ideal management for all is unobtainable, but with sensible use of resources it is possible to treat people in a way that is near to the ideal.

The topic of this presentation is related not to *saving* money but to how we can make the most of the cardiac care budget. Some suggestions may entail greater spending and perhaps some of them reduced spending. The objective then is value and not economy in the sense of spending less. Since logistics are more important to costs than the therapy, these may benefit most from review.

Early treatment
What is our advice about the timing of admission to the cardiac care unit? There is no controversy about this; the idea is to get people in as soon as practicable. There is much more debate about how this can be achieved. At the Royal Sussex County Hospital, the public are asked to notify the hospital within ten minutes of any unusual pain. Instruction has been given to over 40,000 members of the community on what cardiac pain feels like. Unfortunately, education and even the experience of having had an attack are of limited value. People are reluctant to 'bother' the hospital and people are also incredibly optimistic. Interestingly, away-from-home emergencies elicit the quickest response. It is fair to say, however, that strategies for admitting people quickly are not yet very successful. We have to seek ways of doing it better. If earlier admission is achieved then that itself will increase the cost because some who would die from early ventricular fibrillation would then survive to use hospital resources. Also public education programmes do result in some patients presenting at the hospital who do not have cardiac pain.

How can early admissions be achieved? In Brighton, use of the emergency 999 system is encouraged and the general practitioners, when circularized some years ago, were in favour of this. Unfortunately, still only around half of patients use the 999 system.

Ideally a general practitioner should be in attendance as well as the ambulance, but this is rare. It would be ideal if ambulances carried doctors but that, of course, is beyond our resources. Certainly, though, there must be resuscitation facilities in the ambulance, and in particular a defibrillator.

If it is not practicable to carry a doctor in the ambulance, a para-medic is an acceptable compromise. Indeed, an ambulanceman without extended training but able to use an automatic defibrillator can help to save many patients with early ventricular fibrillation. Instruction in the use of an automatic defibrillator requires little time. Policemen at Victoria station, who knew little about first aid, were trained within around two hours. Pre-hospital care, if using ambulances with either para-medics or ambulancemen, can therefore be provided at very modest cost. All ambulances carrying patients with myocardial infarction should be provided with a simple defibrillator, even though this may involve a small capital outlay.

Admission to hospital
Which patients should be admitted? If a speedy response is encouraged by using the 999 system, then the patient filtering process carried out by the general practitioner is lost, resulting in an added burden for the emergency department. The position is especially difficult in these days of scarce resources because it has become very difficult to find empty beds for emergency admissions. This dilemma is not helped by the Medical Defence Union's advice that anybody with possible cardiac pain should be kept in an observation ward overnight. This is not always possible nor even desirable, but this emphasis on defensive medicine adds to the pressure. There is then an increased work-load for cardiac wards and — inevitably — increased cost.

The economical use of a CCU
Where do we arrange the admissions? It is important to remember that there is no safe coronary patient in the first few hours after a myocardial infarction; it is not possible to tell in the first four hours which patient will develop ventricular fibrillation. The cardiac care unit is therefore mandatory for a few hours for most patients. After the first four hours, primary ventricular fibrillation unassociated with failure or shock is extremely uncommon. There is no need to keep patients in the cardiac care unit for 48 hours. Moreover, it is valuable to have a cardiac care unit adjacent to an intensive care unit because that can economize on staff. In the vast majority of cases, the cardiac care unit does little more than provide hotel care. The full facilities of this unit are required only to cope with the occasional emergency. If there is an adjacent high-dependency area any brief requirement for additional staff can readily be met.

General medical wards for convalescent patients
In Brighton, it has been found that it is a safe policy to use open wards for patients with myocardial infarction once the first few critical hours have passed. The resuscitation rates on the open wards are about the same as in the cardiac care unit. When a hospital has an efficient cardiac care unit the training rubs off onto staff nurses and sisters throughout the hospital. Every ward should have a defibrillator. Dr Cobbe has referred to the need for intermediate wards with monitoring (see page 143). I believe that after the first few hours, an ordinary ward with adequate equipment and trained staff will perform just as efficiently. I also believe that the standard recommendation for cardiac care unit beds of 4 per 100,000 population is unnecessarily generous, and that savings can be made here.

The duration of hospital admission
What about the duration of admission? Stratification of risk is not difficult after patients have been admitted to hospital. At Brighton, the low risk group is discharged at four to six days (median five days); patients can easily be selected for whom discharge at four days does not pose any additional risk.

The need for secondary prevention
Stratification of risk can also be used to determine the need for secondary prevention — why burden the low-risk patient with beta-blockers if they are not necessary? Slightly over 30% of our patients are classified as low-risk. When 97 patients were followed prospectively for two years, we observed a zero mortality in this group. Early

complications are also somewhat less common after thrombolysis.

What follows after admission? Routine clinic visits are desirable but not essential. Treadmill testing coupled with a good rehabilitation programme will identify problem patients who ought to attend the clinic. Most hospital follow-up is unnecessary and routine patient evaluation six months after discharge is not required. However, a rehabilitation programme — which is not expensive — is essential.

Conclusion

If the coronary care system is based on the natural history of the disease, savings may not be made overall but the hospital can at least make the most of its budget. The requirements for good cardiac care are, in fact, relatively modest.

Index

Flecainide, 142
Foam cells
  and plaque fissuring, 11
Free fatty acids
  and arrhythmogenesis, 55-9
Free radicals
  and myocardial stunning, 53-4
  and pathophysiology of tissue injury, 51-4
  production during reperfusion, 52
  and reperfusion arrhythmias, 53

General practitioner
  role of, 133-9, 144-5, 149-50
German/Austrian Multi-Centre Clinical Trial,
  103, 105-6
GISSI, 81, 98, 134
GISSI-I, 86
GISSI-II, 66, 92, 98
Glyceryl trinitrate, 88-9
Glycoprotein receptor IIb-IIIa
  monoclonal antibodies to, 20

Haemodynamic parameters, 49
Haemostasis
  in Q-wave infarction, 18
Heparin, 3, 75, 90, 98, 100-3, 106-7, 114-7, 121
Hirudin, 19, 107
Histamine, 30
Hjärta-Smärta-90,000, 131-3
Hypertension
  as a risk factor, 85-6

Implantable defibrillators, 157
Infarct expansion, 59-65
Infarct extension, 59-65
Infarct-related artery
  patency and prognosis, 71-4, 76-7, 118, 120
Infarct size
  factors determining, 4-6, 49-50, 72
  measurement, 45-51
Interleukin 1, 24
International Anticoagulant Review Group, 105
Interuniversity Cardiology Institute of the
  Netherlands, 116
ISAM Study, 69, 72
ISIS-I Study, 84-6, 88-95
ISIS-II Study, 67, 76, 81, 86, 90-1, 96-8, 125,
  127, 129
ISIS-III Study, 66, 98
Isosorbide dinitrate, 29-30, 80, 94

Johns-Hopkins Trial, 112

Ketanserin, 30

Lactate dehydrogenase
  and diagnosis, 46
Left ventricular function
  with thrombolytic therapy, 71-3, 76-9, 85,
  120, 123
Lignocaine, 141-2, 149
Long-term survival
  with thrombolytic therapy, 74, 76
  with thrombolytic therapy and PTCA, 117,
  119-20

Macrophages
  and plaque fissuring, 11, 14, 24-5
Magnesium, 141-2
Magnetic resonance imaging, 38-42
Marker proteins see also: *Creatine kinase*, 82-3
Mast cells, 26
Medical Research Council, 100, 103-4
Methylergonovine, 30
MIAMI Trial, 84, 92
Mobile coronary care units, 127-30
Monoclonal antibodies, 20
Morbidity
  with anticoagulants, 99-110
  with thrombolytic therapy, 66-9
Mortality causes, 84-6, 101-3
Mortality rates
  with antiarrhythmic drugs, 142
  with anticoagulants, 99-110
  with antiplatelet agents, 96-8
  with beta-blockers, calcium antagonists and
  nitrates, 87-95
  and infarct extension, 59
  with thrombolytic therapy, 66-9, 73-4, 76-7, 86,
  90-8, 118-9, 123, 127
  with thrombolytic therapy and PTCA, 113-4,
  117, 119
Myocardial infarction
  diagnosis, 44
  and free fatty acids, 55
  and free radicals, 53
  pathophysiology, 1-9, 12-13, 15, 26, 29, 31
  and ventricular fibrillation, 140-1
Myocardial ischaemia
  diagnosis, 33-65
  and free radical production, 53
  pathophysiology, 1-32
  and ventricular fibrillation, 140
Myocardial necrosis, 18
  non-invasive markers, 33-7
Myocardial oxygen demand
  in unstable angina, 18
Myocardial salvage
  and PTCA, 112
Myocardial stunning, 53-4
Myoglobin, 82-3
Myosin light chains, 35-6, 82-3

Neuropeptide Y, 31
Nifedipine, 88-9
Nitrates, 16, 30, 87-95, 149
Nitroglycerin, 79
Non-invasive indices of thrombolysis, 81-3
Non-Q-wave infarction
  pathophysiology, 4, 6, 17-18

Opiates, 148-9
Oxygen radicals see: *Free radicals*

Pain relief, 148-9
Patency rates
  with thrombolysis, 71, 111, 122-3
  with thrombolysis and PTCA, 115-7
Patient selection, 81-3, 128, 132-3, 146, 159
Percutaneous transluminal coronary angioplasty
  after thrombolysis, 111-21
Phenindione, 100, 102, 104
Phenotolamine, 30